The Attachment-Based Compassion Therapy

Javier García-Campayo • Daniel Campos
Paola Herrera-Mercadal • Mayte Navarro-Gil
Kathryn Ziemer • Beatriz Palma
Sheeva Mostoufi • Roberto Aristegui

The Attachment-Based Compassion Therapy

A Manual for Self-Application

Springer

Javier García-Campayo
School of Medicine
University of Zaragoza
Zaragoza, Zaragoza, Spain

Paola Herrera-Mercadal
Department of Psychology and Sociology
University of Zaragoza
Zaragoza, Zaragoza, Spain

Kathryn Ziemer
Old Town Psychology
Alexandria, VA, USA

Sheeva Mostoufi
Old Town Psychology
Alexandria, VA, USA

Daniel Campos
Department of Psychology and Sociology
University of Zaragoza
Zaragoza, Zaragoza, Spain

Mayte Navarro-Gil
Department of Psychology and Sociology
University of Zaragoza
Zaragoza, Zaragoza, Spain

Beatriz Palma
Counseling And Psychological Services
University of Virginia
Charlottesville, VA, USA

Roberto Aristegui
School of Psychology
Adolfo Ibáñez University
Santiago, RM - Santiago, Chile

ISBN 978-3-031-38031-0 ISBN 978-3-031-38032-7 (eBook)
https://doi.org/10.1007/978-3-031-38032-7

This Springer imprint is published by the registered company Springer Nature Switzerland AG
The registered company address is: Gewerbestrasse 11, 6330 Cham, Switzerland

Acknowledgments

The authors thank Pilar Iñigo Gias for the photographs.

Contents

List of Figures

List of Tables

List of Practices

About the Authors

Javier García-Campayo practices psychiatry at Hospital Universitario Miguel Servet, in Zaragoza, Spain. He is professor at the University of Zaragoza School of Medicine and director of the Master's degree program in Mindfulness and the Chair of Contemplative Science at the same institution. Dr García-Campayo graduated in Medicine and obtained his PhD in Psychiatry from the University of Zaragoza. He is a former president of the Spanish Society of Psychosomatic Medicine.

Daniel Campos holds the position of assistant professor in the Department of Psychology and Sociology (Sub-Department of Developmental Psychology and Education) at the University of Zaragoza, Spain, and is a member of the master's degree program in Mindfulness at the same institution. Dr Campos graduated in Psychology and obtained his PhD and master's degree in Psychopathology, Health, and Neuropsychology from the Universitat Jaume I (Castellón, Spain). He was awarded a post-doctoral grant to develop the project entitled Compassion Therapy for Well-being: Development of an Online Intervention. He has worked on several projects financed by local, national, and international research grants focusing on the application of information and communication technologies (ICTs), mindfulness, and compassion-based Interventions.

Paola Herrera-Mercadal is lecturer in the Department of Psychology and Sociology (Sub-Department of Developmental Psychology and Education) at the University of Zaragoza, Spain, and a member of the master's degree program in Mindfulness at the same institution. Dr Herrera-Mercadal graduated in Psychology from the National University of Distance Education (UNED) of Spain and obtained both a master's degree in Introduction to Medical Research and her PhD in Medicine from the Universidad of Zaragoza. She has worked on several projects financed by local, national, and international research grants focusing on the application of ICTs, mindfulness, and compassion-based interventions.

Mayte Navarro-Gil graduated in Psychology from the National University of Distance Education (UNED) of Spain. She obtained her PhD in Medicine specializing in mindfulness and compassion. She has published different articles on this topic and is a mindfulness instructor with extensive experience in teaching, clinical application, and research in this technique. She is currently lecturer in the Department of Psychology and Sociology at the University of Zaragoza, and teaches part of the program for the master's degree in Mindfulness at the same institution.

Kathryn Ziemer is a licensed psychologist and the Clinical Director at Old Town Psychology, a psychology practice that provides evidence-based therapy and conducts applied research. She received her PhD from the University of Maryland and completed her internship at the DC Veterans Affairs Medical Center. She has conducted research at the US National Institute of Mental Health, the Social and Decision Analytics Lab at Virginia Polytechnic Institute and State University, and the market research company Ipsos Public Affairs. Her research interests include attachment, self-compassion, meaning in life, brief psychological interventions, intersection of technology and mental health, and the promotion of positive psychology. She has over ten years' experience providing psychological services, including evidence-based therapy, to clients experiencing depression, anxiety, chronic health conditions, infertility, relationship issues, and life transitions. She has previously provided psychological services at the University of Maryland Counseling Center and the George Mason University Cognitive Assessment Program.

Beatriz Palma is a licensed psychologist and group coordinator at Counseling and Psychological Services (CAPS) at the University of Virginia (UVA) – Charlottesville. She earned her bachelor's degree in Psychology and Psychologist Professional Degree from Pontificia Universidad Católica de Chile. After working as a clinical psychologist in Chile for five years, she moved to the United States and earned an MEd from Penn State and an MS and PhD from the University of Maryland – College Park. Her research interests include attachment, self-compassion, the therapeutic relationship, psychotherapy process and outcome, supervision and training, and group therapy. In the United States, she has provided psychological services in several university settings, including the Counseling Center at the University of Missouri – Columbia, where she completed a Post Internship/Postdoctoral Psychology Residency. She also provided long-term, psychodynamic-oriented individual therapy to adults in the community at the Maryland Psychotherapy Clinic and Research Lab (MPCRL). Her areas of clinical specialty include trauma, family of origin issues, multicultural and intercultural issues, identities and intersectionality, and group therapy. She also served as the Early Career Psychologist – Domain Representative from the Society for the Advancement of Psychotherapy from the American Psychological Association (APA) from 2020 to 2022.

Sheeva Mostoufi is a licensed clinical psychologist and training coordinator at Old Town Psychology, a psychology practice that provides evidence-based psychotherapy and conducts applied research. She received her PhD from the San Diego State University/University of California, San Diego Joint Doctoral Program and completed her internship at the VA Puget Sound Health Care System-Seattle Division. She also completed postdoctoral fellowship training at the VA Puget Sound Health Care System-Seattle Division specializing in primary care mental health integration. She has conducted research on grant-funded research studies with the US Veteran Affairs Health Care System and with the community-based University of Washington Twin Registry. She has a background in clinical research with multiple publications in peer-reviewed journals. Her research interests include self-compassion, mindfulness-based interventions, culturally affirming delivery of evidence-based treatments, and mechanisms of change in clinical interventions. She specializes in treating clients presenting with obsessive compulsive disorder (OCD), social anxiety, generalized anxiety disorder, body-focused repetitive behaviors (e.g., trichotillomania, excoriation/skin picking), depression, life transitions, and coping with chronic medical concerns. She has experience providing evidence-based psychotherapies such as Acceptance and Commitment Therapy and Exposure and Response Prevention to clients in a variety of settings, including private practice, as a clinician on grant-funded research studies with the Veteran Affairs Health Care System, and in interdisciplinary hospital and medical settings.

Roberto Aristegui is a clinical psychologist specializing in Psychotherapy. He is an assistant professor in the Department of Psychiatry and Mental Health at the University of Chile, where he co-directs a diploma in mindfulness and relational skills. As an adjunct professor at the Faculty of Psychology of the Adolfo Ibáñez University, he is the director of the master's degree in Relational Mindfulness and Compassion at that institution. He has a degree in Psychology from the Catholic University of Chile and a PhD in Philosophy from the University of Chile. He has participated in projects funded by local, national, and international research grants and currently in the relational approach. He has a PhD in Social Sciences from Tilburg University, the Netherlands, where he worked with Kenneth Gergen on social constructionism, promoting the Relational Mindfulness perspective.

Abbreviations

ABCT	Attachment-Based Compassion Therapy
CBCT	Cognitive-Based Compassion Therapy
CBIs	Compassion-Based Interventions
CCT	Compassion Cultivation Training
CFT	Compassion Focused Therapy
DIY	Do It yourself
MSC	Mindful Self-Compassion

Chapter 1
Introduction to the Book and Recommendations for Its Use

1 The Attachment-Based Compassion Therapy: Conceptualization and Evidence to Date

Compassion has been described as a psychological process that involves recognizing suffering in oneself (self-compassion) or another person, viewing that suffering as part of the shared human experience, connecting with the emotions of others, tolerating any distress, and experiencing motivation to help (Gu et al., 2020; Strauss et al., 2016).

Compassion therapy is a third-generation psychotherapy that has been used in association with mindfulness in recent years. Recently developed compassion-based interventions (CBIs) explicitly focusing on cultivating compassion and self-compassion have yielded promising results for increasing compassion toward self and others and to promote both health-related and well-being outcomes, in the general population, and have been shown to effectively treat of a number of different psychological disorders (Austin et al., 2021; Kirby et al., 2017; Millard et al., 2023; Wakelin et al., 2022). Research has related increased compassion to reduced depressive (Krieger et al., 2016; López et al., 2018; Raes et al., 2011), anxiety (Blackie & Kocovski, 2018; Werner et al., 2012), and stress symptoms (Allen & Leary, 2010; Dahm et al., 2015; Hu et al., 2018), among other mental health outcomes. Studies have pointed out that compassion might impact mental health by facilitating adaptive emotion regulation (Inwood & Ferrari, 2018) and reducing self-criticism (Wakelin et al., 2022). However, compassion (and self-compassion) is associated not only with reduced psychopathology but also with a range of adaptive and prosocial variables, such as happiness (Campos et al., 2016; Pandey et al., 2021), satisfaction with life (Yang et al., 2016), and well-being (Neff, 2011; Zessin et al., 2015), as well as with the promotion of physical health and healthy behaviors (Phillips & Hine, 2021).

J. García-Campayo et al., *The Attachment-Based Compassion Therapy*,
https://doi.org/10.1007/978-3-031-38032-7_1

In particular, attachment-based compassion therapy (ABCT) is a protocol that aims to promote compassion and self-compassion in both the general and clinical psychiatric populations (García-Campayo & Demarzo, 2015; García-Campayo et al., 2016a, b). In the face-to-face group format, ABCT has demonstrated efficacy, applicability, and cost-utility for healthy people and for individuals diagnosed with fibromyalgia, depression, anxiety, and adjustment disorders from Spain (e.g., Collado-Navarro et al., 2021; D'Amico et al., 2020; Montero-Marín et al., 2018, 2019; Navarro-Gil et al., 2018; Lopez-del-Hoyo et al., 2022). Moreover, ABCT seems to reduce brain-derived neurotrophic factor and appears to have anti-inflammatory effects in fibromyalgia patients (Montero-Marin et al., 2019). Navarro-Gil et al. (2018) found that ABCT promoted self-compassion, and mindfulness as well as reduced psychological distress, anxiety, and avoidance in healthy individuals. In addition, secure attachment style significantly increased after completing ABCT and was mediated by changes in self-compassion. This indicates that ABCT may be an effective intervention for improving compassion and secure attachment style in healthy adults in the general populations.

ABCT is based on attachment theory and, therefore, includes practices to raise awareness of the attachment styles individuals have with their parents and to address any maladaptive aspects of the relationship with themselves and others. This process is taught as a form of both compassion and self-compassion in order to improve present-day interpersonal relationships and well-being in general. As with other compassion protocols, ABCT has incorporated a number of practices and theoretical foundations based on traditions such as Tibetan Buddhism but also from other religions and belief systems in which compassion plays a part, given that it is the common denominator in all of them. For this intervention, as is typical in mindfulness and compassion-based therapies, any religious or cultural connotation has been removed from these techniques, and their efficacy has been evaluated from a scientific perspective.

2 Information on the Self-Applied Attachment-Based Compassion Therapy and the Structure of the Book

This book consists of an adapted version of ABCT that can be self-applied by any individual in a psychoeducational context or as a support for therapy guided by a professional in order to promote secure attachment through compassion and increased understanding of the suffering in oneself and in others. This protocol aims to help people improve their own well-being and that of others.

The self-applied version of the ABCT operates along the lines of the original model and has been adapted and developed to be fully self-applied via the Internet (Campos et al., 2020), and this manual for self-application has been designed for use as bibliotherapy and psychoeducational material. The ABCT protocol described in this book has been translated from Spanish into English by the authors of this manual and future research is planed using the online version.

This version consists of seven sequential modules, each with the same structure: (1) objectives, (2) theoretical contents of the module, (3) exercises and activities (including formal and informal practices) that enable the contents of the module to be put into practice, (4) assessment of the knowledge acquired during the module, (5) series of tasks to be completed before advancing to the next module (homework assignments), (6) annexes, and (7) summary of the module.

The content is presented through text, pictures, tables, and figures, including links to downloadable audio files for formal meditation practices with specific guides and instructions for each meditation. The transcripts to each guided meditation are also included as appendices.

In comparison with the original ABCT, the adapted version for self-application includes Module 0, "Introduction to attachment-based compassion therapy," to introduce participants to the basics of the attachment-based compassion model and the program contents. Module 0 also includes practical advice on the use of formal and informal compassion exercises (when/where/how much/how to meditate) and on the importance of consistency in compassion training and of home practice between modules. Specific content has been added about "managing guilt" (formal meditation in Module 4), "shame" (theoretical component and formal practice in Module 5), and "envy" (theoretical component and formal practice in Module 7). Moreover, the term "the figure of affect" has been replaced with "basic affection" for ease of understanding and to avoid confusion with "the figure of secure attachment." Other practices that have been eliminated are "Showing forgiveness for the hurt caused by loved ones" (for people with grief experiences) and the "The illusion of labels" because they were not considered relevant for this ABCT version. Finally, Module 8 on equanimity ("Beyond compassion: equanimity") (García-Campayo et al., 2016a, b) has not been included in the self-applied version because it was considered a distinct and more advanced aspect of compassion.

The manual of ABCT for self-application is structured in nine chapters. This chapter, "Introduction to the Book and Recommendations for Its Use," includes basic information on the structure of the book and provides recommendations and advice on how to use the manual and how to adapt it to particular teaching contexts (e.g., clinical or psychoeducational). This chapter also includes an explanation regarding how not to use the manual. Chapters 2, 3, 4, 5, 6, 7, 8 and 9 are the modules of the self-application version of the ABCT. A glossary is included at the end with meanings or definitions of special, unusual, or technical words or phrases that has been mentioned throughout the manual.

Chapter 2: Module 0: Understanding Attachment-Based Compassion Therapy

Module 0 introduces readers to the basics of the model, and the following theoretical components are explained and put into practice: what compassion is, contexts of application, structure of and rationale behind attachment-based compassion therapy, and meditation and compassion (formal and informal practice). It also offers practical advice on the practice of meditation (when/where/how much/how to meditate) and explains the importance of working into compassion and when doing homework. Instructions on how to perform the "3 compassionate minutes" practice are also provided.

Chapter 3: Module 1: Preparing Ourselves for Compassion: Kind Attention

Module 1 focuses on how our brain works, the reality of suffering, the difference between primary and secondary suffering, and what compassion is and is not. The formal practices "Compassionate breathing and compassionate body scan" and "Compassionate coping with difficulties" are implemented and explained in Module 1. The module also explains the self-compassion journal and introduces the exercise "Gratitude" as an informal practice.

Chapter 4: Module 2: Discovering Our Compassionate World

Module 2 includes the following theoretical components: a deeper understanding of compassion and mindfulness terms, compassion and related terms, and concerns about compassion. The formal practices included are "Connecting with basic affection," "Developing a safe place," "The compassionate gesture," and "Identify the attachment figure." Recommended informal practices for Module 2 are "The object that connects you to the world," "Compassion practice journal," and the exercise "What are you good at?"

Chapter 5: Module 3: Developing our Compassionate World

Module 3 provides information on how compassion works, the figure of secure attachment, efficacy of compassion, and self-criticism. This content is implemented through the practices "Developing the attachment figure," "Replacing the critical voice with the compassionate voice," and "Letter from the attachment figure."

Chapter 6: Module 4: Understanding Our Relationship with Compassion

Module 4 provides readers with information regarding the biological foundations of compassion, attachment patterns, guilt, and the importance of attachment patterns in daily life. The formal practices introduced in the module are "Become aware of our attachment pattern," "Capacity to receive affection (friend, neutral people, and enemies)," and "Repairing guilt." Finally, the module will include "Letter to parents or caregivers" and the exercise "Observe how the attachment patterns show up in daily life" as informal practice.

Chapter 7: Module 5: Working on Ourselves

The importance of the affection we have toward ourselves and others and shame are the main contents of Module 5. A guide is provided to the following formal practices: "Give affection to friends and neutral people," "Giving ourselves affection," "Reconciling with parental figures," and "Repairing shame." The informal practices included in Module 5 are "The greatest show of affection ever received" and "Three positive and three negative things about your parental figures."

Chapter 8: Module 6: Understanding the Importance of Forgiveness

Module 6 focuses on the following topics in order to facilitate understanding of the importance of forgiveness: the concept of forgiveness, phases of forgiveness, utility of forgiveness, basic forms of barriers to generating forgiveness, resources for generating forgiveness, and recapitulation (optional). The formal meditations that enable these theoretical components to be put into practice are "Forgiving yourself," "Asking others for forgiveness," and "Forgive others and give compassion to enemies." The "Interdependence" practice and "Compassion in daily life" exercises are provided as informal practice.

Chapter 9: Module 7: Consolidating the Practice of Compassion

The final module includes information on the importance of working in three perspectives (past, present, and future), envy, the usefulness of being our own attachment figure, difficulties in relationships, and how to keep up the practice of compassion throughout life. The formal practices provided in Module 7 are

"Working with envy and developing joy for the success of others," "Becoming our own attachment figure," and "Managing emotions that could create challenges in relationships." The informal practices included are "Changing your perspective," "Our values and their relation to compassion," and "What would our life be like if we started over?"

3 Recommendations on How to Use the Manual

As we mentioned above, this manual can be used by any individual in a psychoeducational context or as a support for a therapeutic process guided by a professional. In cases of personal use, we recommend completion of one module per week, with the days between sessions used to complete homework assignments. Readers can find basic information in the text of each module and additional content in the annexes to go deeper according to their needs. For meditations, both audios and their transcripts are provided, so that the reader can choose how to practice them. Initially, we recommend following guided meditation according to the frequency outlined in the modules. Expert meditators can perform meditations in silence, guiding themselves and based on the content of each meditation.

Notes regarding mandatory and additional (or voluntary) content are included throughout. Nevertheless, we recommend that readers be aware of their needs at the time in their life that they're using this self-applied manual. Given that these meditations may elicit difficult emotions, we encourage readers to pick and choose which practices best fit with their individual needs. It is not strictly necessary to practice all the content included, or all at once. We invite readers to take this as an opportunity to understand and know themselves a little better. Compassion (and self-compassion) should be like a mattress where you can rest and prepare for action.

Each module has been optimized to allow it to be completed in approximately 1 hour. We estimate that the self-applied protocol can be completed in 8 to 10 weeks. However, readers are free to advance at their own pace, spending the time that they need to practice and consolidate the content of one module before advancing to the next. It is important to take into account that the original ABCT protocol is delivered in weekly sessions for 8 weeks, reporting a notable adherence to the intervention (i.e., 81.5% of sessions attended, on average) (Montero-Marín et al., 2018). However, some adaptations of the program may be helpful for certain groups of participants. For example, ABCT was adapted for fibromyalgia patients who had expressed difficulties in previous studies about remaining seated for long periods of time (i.e., around 2 hours) in psychotherapy sessions and focusing on instructors' explanations due to cognitive difficulties. Therefore, a 16-session version of ABCT was created, and a preliminary study exploring its efficacy found improvements in anxiety and depressive symptomatology in fibromyalgia patients (Santos et al., 2022).

Individuals in need of further psychological assistance are advised to seek professional help that would help them determine how to integrate compassion-based strategies into their therapy work. Physical and mental health professionals who would like to apply these techniques are advised to train themselves in meditation practices. Teacher training for instructors on the ABCT model is delivered via https://terapiadecompasion.com/. Therapists who have received formal training in ABCT can order this manual for their patients to be used as bibliotherapy in a blended format or as a support material.

Regarding how not to use this manual, we do not recommend using it to treat one-self as self-therapy, or as a substitute for professional help when necessary. Specially, people who have suffered abuse and/or other traumatic experiences are advised to seek professional help before engaging in the self-application of the ABCT manual.

Chapter 2
Module 0: Understanding Attachment-Based Compassion Therapy

Module Objectives

In this module, we want to help you achieve the following goals:

- Learn what compassion is.
- Understand the contexts in which compassion is applied and each of its objectives.
- Understand the theoretical bases for the intervention, including attachment theory and compassion meditation.
- Learn how to use meditation, and learn the difference between formal and informal practice.
- Understand how to structure the practice of compassion meditation.
- Reflect on the importance of working into compassion and doing homework.
- Learn the informal practice, "3 Compassionate Minutes" that will allow you to become familiar with compassion in an approachable way.

Go ahead with the module. Don't feel like you need to hurry through it. It's more important to try to understand all the concepts that are presented and practice the exercises.

Module Contents

1. What is Compassion
2. Application Contexts
3. Attachment-Based Compassion Therapy: Explanation and Structure
4. Using Meditation in Compassion: Formal and Informal Practice and Posture
5. General Tips on Practicing Meditation
6. The Importance of Working into Compassion and Homework
7. Informal Practice of 3 Compassionate Minutes

Supplementary Information The online version contains supplementary material available at https://doi.org/10.1007/978-3-031-38032-7_2.

J. García-Campayo et al., *The Attachment-Based Compassion Therapy*,
https://doi.org/10.1007/978-3-031-38032-7_2

8. Self-Assessment Questions
9. Homework
10. Annexes

Welcome! We're glad that you decided to start this journey of self-growth. We strongly suggest that you don't rush to finish the module; take time to review the information and try to understand all the concepts presented and engage in all the practices that are introduced. You will get the most out of this intervention by taking your time with the material.

1 What Is Compassion

Origin of Compassion

The word compassion comes from the Latin word *compati* "to suffer with." Initially, many defined compassion as feeling pity toward someone who's suffering. Definitions of compassion that include the feeling of pity are present even today. For example, Collins online dictionary states "Compassion is a feeling of pity, sympathy, and understanding for someone who is suffering" (https://www.collinsdictionary.com/us/dictionary/english/compassion).

The focus on pity implies feeling superior to the person who is suffering. However, we think about compassion in a very different way in this intervention, because we view it as a feeling between equals.

Compassion in Psychology

Here are some common definition of compassion from psychology:

> A sensitivity to suffering in self and others with a commitment to try to alleviate and prevent it (Paul Gilbert 2015).

> Compassion is a relational process that involves noticing another person's pain, experiencing an emotional reaction to his or her pain, and acting in some way to help ease or alleviate the pain (Kanov et al., 2004).

When compassion is directed toward yourself, it's called self-compassion. Here's the definition of self-compassion:

> Being open to and moved by one's own suffering, experiencing feelings of caring and kindness toward oneself, taking an understanding, nonjudgmental attitude toward one's inadequacies and failures, and recognizing that one's own experience is part of the common human experience (Neff, 2003a, b).

The two key elements of compassion are (Simón, 2014):

- Sensitivity to the suffering of others and of ourselves
- Commitment to alleviate that suffering

Table 2.1 Compassion protocols

Protocol	CBCT	CCT	CFT	MSC
Name	Cognitive-based compassion therapy	Compassion cultivation training	Compassion-focused therapy	Mindful self-compassion
Origin	Lama Tenzin Negi, University of Emory (USA)	Lama Tupten Jinpa, University of Stanford (USA)	Paul Gilbert (Derby University, Britain)	Kristin Neff and Christopher Germer (University of Texas, USA)
Base	Buddhist tradition (Practice of Lo-Jong)	Buddhist tradition (Practice of Lo-Jong)	Western psychology (development of the compassionate self)	Mix of western psychology and Buddhist (based on MBSR and the practice of loving kindness)
Target audience	Patients and healthy populations	Patients and healthy populations	Patients	Patients and healthy populations
Reference	Pace, Negi, et al. (2009)	Jazaieri et al. (2013)	Gilbert (2015)	Neff (2012)

Note. *CBCT* cognitive-based compassion therapy, *CCT* compassion cultivation Training, *CFT* compassion-focused therapy, *MSC* mindful self-compassion

The sensitivity to suffering is based on empathy. This means putting yourself in the other person's shoes and understanding what the other person might be thinking or feeling (i.e., also called "mentalizing" or theory of mind).

A key part of compassion is the desire to alleviate the pain of others. That is why compassion is a motivation (not an emotion) that guides human behavior (Gilbert, 2015).

Compassion-Based Interventions

Compassion-based interventions help people use compassion in everyday life. These interventions are usually structured (e.g., use a manual) and use theory, practice, and exercises to help people develop compassion (and self-compassion).

In Table 2.1 you will find detailed information on the main compassion protocols.

Compassion protocols tend to be structured in 8 weeks, in sessions of 2 or 2 and a half hours, or in intensive courses of 2 or 3 days.

2 Application Contexts

Compassion can be applied in different ways, depending on the context.

1. Clinical Level

   At the clinical level, compassion interventions are used with patients who have a medical or psychiatric diagnosis and who want to treat or improve a specific illness (e.g., depression, anxiety, chronic pain, etc.). In these cases, compassion therapy often follows a manual and is often administered by healthcare professionals.

2. Psychoeducational level
   At the psychoeducational level, compassion interventions are used with the general population. This includes people who do not have any clinical diagnosis and who seek to improve their general health and psychological well-being (e.g., reduce rumination, learn to cope with adverse situations, regulate emotions, etc.). Manuals are also often used (although it is not essential) and can be administered by people trained in therapy, but don't need to be healthcare professionals. The interventions may be aimed at specific groups such as students in schools or universities or professionals in organizations.
3. Spiritual level
4. At the spiritual level, compassion interventions are used with people (healthy or not) who are pursuing spiritual development and transcendence. The use of compassion in this context usually doesn't follow structured and concise manuals (although they could be used) but instead follows the norms of a specific religious tradition. It's usually taught by spiritual teachers or people with recognized experience in meditation and who have certain ethical principles and values.

3 Attachment-Based Compassion Therapy: Explanation and Structure

Attachment-based compassion therapy (ABCT) is a compassion-based intervention developed in Spain by the research group of Dr. Javier García-Campayo (https://www.webmindfulness.com/; https://www.javiergarciacampayo.com/)

This intervention is based on attachment theory and the use of compassion meditation, two methods that have shown to improve psychological well-being. This is one of the first interventions to combine the known theory and research on both attachment and compassion into a self-guided program for the purpose of improving psychological health, relationships, and overall well-being.

Specifically, the intervention is based on the following:

1. Attachment theory: Attachment theory explains the way we relate to ourselves and to other people. There are different patterns of attachment, which influence how we manage our emotions with ourselves and others. Knowing your attachment pattern and changing the unhelpful parts can reduce stress in your life. This intervention is meant to help you develop a secure attachment pattern, which can lower criticism and anger toward yourself and others and increase compassion.
2. Contributions of religious/spiritual tradition: Like other compassion interventions, some practices and theories in this intervention come from Tibetan Buddhism, as well as other religions based in compassion. For this intervention,

any religious or cultural connotations have been removed, and we focus on the parts of the intervention that have been scientifically proven to be effective.

3. Contributions of other models of compassion and other therapies: This intervention includes ideas from other compassion interventions (e.g., Paul Gilbert's structure of the three brain circuits), as well as techniques from other type of therapy (e.g., mindfulness, acceptance and commitment therapy, dialectical behavioral therapy).

Structure of Internet Attachment-Based Compassion Therapy (iABCT)

This program is an online version of the ABCT that has been adapted and optimized for online use.

The intervention consists of eight modules that are completely self-guided. Each module takes between 60 and 90 minutes to complete and includes text, images, illustrations, videos, audios with guided meditations, exercises, and homework.

The 8 modules are:

Module 0. Understanding Attachment-Based Compassion Therapy
Module 1. Preparing for Compassion: Kind Attention
Module 2. Discovering Our Compassionate World
Module 3. Developing Our Compassionate World
Module 4. Understanding Our Relationship with Compassion
Module 5. Working on Ourselves
Module 6. Understanding the Importance of Forgiveness
Module 7. Consolidating the Practice of Compassion

We recommend doing one module a week and using the time between modules to do the homework. However, you can follow the schedule that best suits you, but we recommend you complete the eight modules in a maximum of 10 weeks. Even if you do one module a week, you don't have to finish it all at once. You can go back to the module as many times as you need, but we recommend that you reserve a time of day when you have time to complete the module without distractions or interruptions.

In the annexes we present an outline of the structure and content of ABCT for self-application.

4 Using Mindfulness and Meditation: Informal and Formal Practice and Posture

Mindfulness is the act of consciously focusing the mind on the present moment, being aware of any thoughts, emotions, or sensations that arise for you. If you find yourself judging yourself, just notice it and let it pass.

Mindfulness is the opposite of automatic, habitual, or rote behavior and activity. When mindful, we are alert and awake, actively observing everything in our environment.

Mindfulness doesn't mean rigidly clinging to the present moment, as if clinging hard enough would keep the present moment from changing. When mindful, we are open to the fluidity of each moment as it arises and falls away. Each moment is a new beginning, a new and unique moment in time.

Mindfulness also doesn't mean rejecting, suppressing, blocking, or avoiding the present moment. Instead, when we're mindful, we enter into each moment (Linehan, 2014).

There are different definitions of meditation based on different traditions. For example, in Zen Buddhism, there's the practice of "watching your mind." In other traditions, you may be asked to focus your mind on specific words or images. The exercises in our intervention are secular and include both focusing on specific words/images (e.g., attachment figure) as well as watching your mind, or contemplating something while sitting or standing quietly for a period of time (Linehan, 2014). According to the Dahl et al. (2015), compassion-based meditations are categorized into the constructive family based on its primary cognitive mechanism.

In this intervention, meditation is used as a tool to help you learn and use compassion. Specifically, we use meditation in both formal and informal practice.

The Difference Between Formal and Informal Practice

Formal practice involves selecting a specific predetermined place and time to practice/meditate (e.g., Tuesdays and Thursdays from 8:00p.m. to 8:30p.m.), and using a specific practice or technique (e.g., compassionate breathing, compassionate body scan, etc.).

On the other hand, informal practice does not have a specific time but is carried out at any time of the day or during downtime (e.g., in line at the supermarket, in the

Table 2.2 Examples of times to do information practice

Examples of times to do information practice
Care and grooming: brushing teeth, showering/bathing, performing physiological needs, washing hands, shaving, combing, cutting hair
Food: buying food, cooking, washing, eating
Maintenance of clothes (washing, ironing, sewing) and of the house (cleaning, making beds, DIY, taking care of the garden or plants)
Commuting: walking, driving, taking the train/bus/metro, climbing stairs, taking the elevator
Dead times that require waiting: traffic jam, appointments (e.g., doctor, lawyer, etc.), line at public services or supermarkets, hotel reception, red lights, etc.

DIY do it yourself

bathroom, on the street, etc.), during day-to-day activities but with a particular attitude of attention and kindness.

The following Table 2.2 summarizes the times of the day that could be times to engage in informal practice.

During the routine activities, instead of thinking about what you did yesterday or what you will do tomorrow, daydreaming, or rushing to finish some activity, you can do an active meditation practice, as described in the box below:

> Become aware of your breathing and your body movements, discovering how every second, even if you are doing the same thing, is different. In this way, you will get to enjoy activities that may have seemed tremendously boring and uncreative.

5 General Advice on the Practice of Meditation

Where to Meditate?

- Quiet place, not noisy (as far as possible), that you are comfortable, with few distractions.
- Comfortable temperature, neither cold nor hot.
- Dim lighting, it should not be excessive or in the dark.
- Create routines by choosing the same place of meditation (if possible).
- Include the use of accessories to create a relaxing atmosphere (e.g., candles, meditation bells, inspiring image, etc.).

When to Meditate?

- Structure your time and reserve a fixed time in your schedule for formal practices.
- The best moments of the usually day tend to be (1) the start of the day because you have a fresh mind and where the effects of meditation can spread throughout

the day and evening or (2) end of the day (e.g., before dinner or before going to the bed) when you can focus on the present and let the worries of the day go. The time of day that works best depends on each person, their preferences, needs, and work situation.
- Remember that meditating at any time of the day, even if unexpected, is better than not meditating.

How Much to Meditate?

- Start for short periods, such as 5 to 10 minutes, and gradually increase it over time.
- At first, it's better to have short meditations more often.
- Consistency is the key. Performing practices on a daily and regular basis produces greater benefits than intense and sporadic practices.
- For the times when you are not meditating with audios or recorded practices, we recommend that you use an alarm clock that alerts you when to start and end your practices.

How to Meditate?

Attitude

- Openness and curiosity to the experience.
- Put aside expectations and observe what happens in the mind.
- End the meditation with the commitment to carry out what is practiced in daily life.

Posture

Posture is a key aspect of meditation practice. This should be comfortable and one that does not cause discomfort but at the same time does not produce excessive relaxation or induce sleep.

The most comfortable postures are usually sitting in a chair or lying on the floor. You can also adopt other typical yoga or meditation postures, although this is not at all necessary.

Following we add some content to expand the information on the different meditation postures. Depending on your needs, you can read and practice them or go ahead with this module.

The two most comfortable and frequent meditation postures are the following:

1. Sitting on a chair: Remember that the chair must be normal and ideally without armrests. We don't recommend leaning your back on the backrest because it tends to sag. You'll want to make sure that the soles of your feet are well supported on the ground and that your chin is slightly dropped. You can rest your

hands on your thighs with your palms up, your fingers intertwined, or touching your index finger and thumb. In all postures, we recommend closing your eyes to avoid distractions, at least in the beginning. When people spend time in meditation, sometimes they prefer a semi-open position of their eyes, looking at a distance between 10 and 15 feet. This is meant to be done in a way that feels natural.

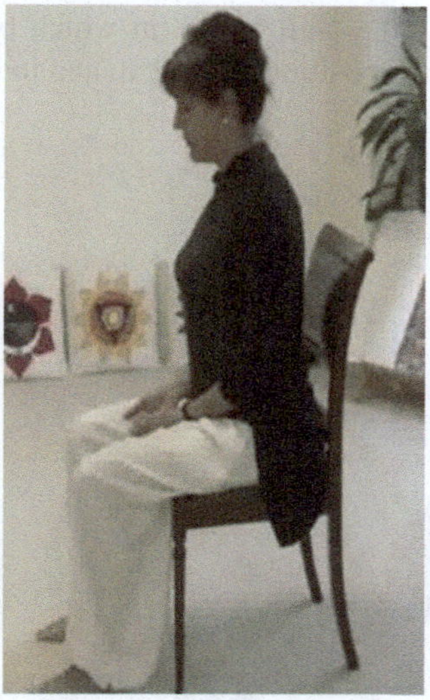

2. Lying on the ground: This position is not usually recommended, except for some practices such as the body scan, since the tendency is to fall asleep. However, it's an option if you cannot do it in any other way. Your neck should be comfortable (you can use a cushion). If you have pain or mobility problems, you can use a cushion under your knees since it tends to be more comfortable and less painful. For pregnant women, we recommend lying on your side, with a cushion to support your face and head and another cushion between your legs, which creates a more comfortable posture.

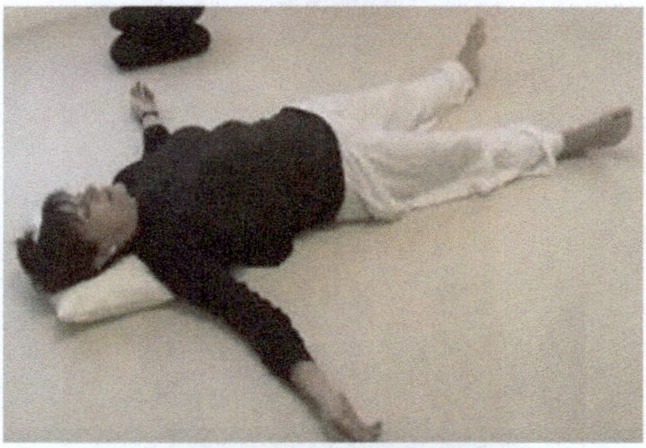

Below are other sitting postures that tend to be a bit more difficult but also suitable for stability when doing meditation. Your posture should be stable and at the same time your back should remain straight to help you stay awake and not fall asleep. In all postures where you're sitting on the floor, we recommend that your hip is higher than your legs, and using a meditation cushion can help with this.

- The best-known form is the "full lotus," in which both feet are on top of the thighs. It is a very difficult position to achieve and to keep.

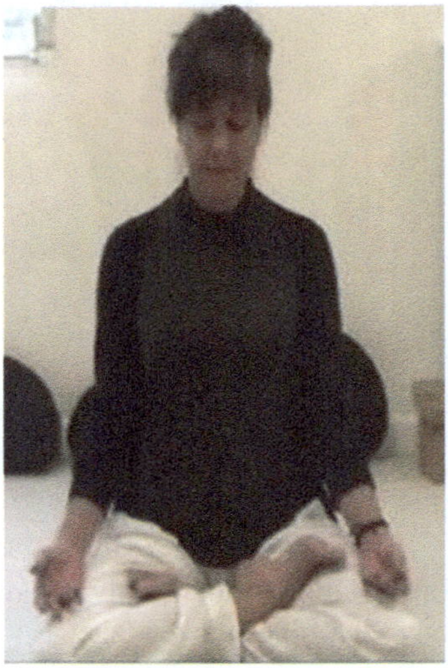

- A more frequent way of sitting for people who already have high meditation experience would be the "half lotus"; it is only one foot that remains above the thigh, and during practice it changes progressively from one side to side.

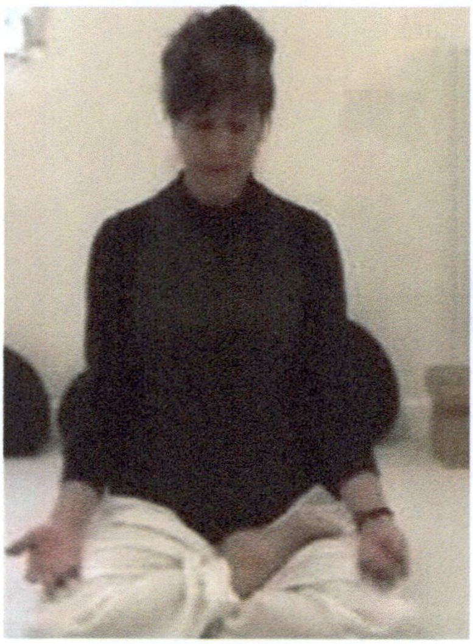

- A simpler and easier posture to maintain would be the "quarter lotus" posture, in which the foot is not placed on the thigh but on the leg and the other foot on the ground. It is a very stable and relatively simple posture.

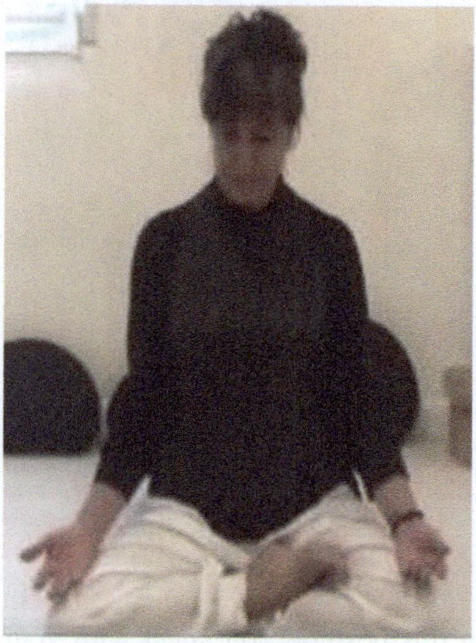

- One of the simplest postures within the "stable postures" would be the "Burmese posture." In it, the feet are placed neither on the thigh nor on the knee but are simply resting on the ground' it is key that your knees touch the ground, providing total stability.

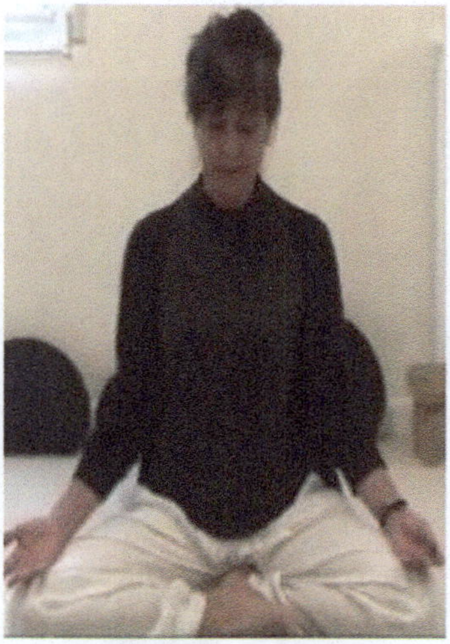

- On the other hand, a position that is not as recommended, although very frequently used, would be cross-legged posture. It is the most comfortable and easy to do. The drawback is that as your knees do not touch the ground the posture is not stable, and it is difficult to maintain beyond 15–20 minutes without pain. For this reason, we recommend using a backrest such as a wall.

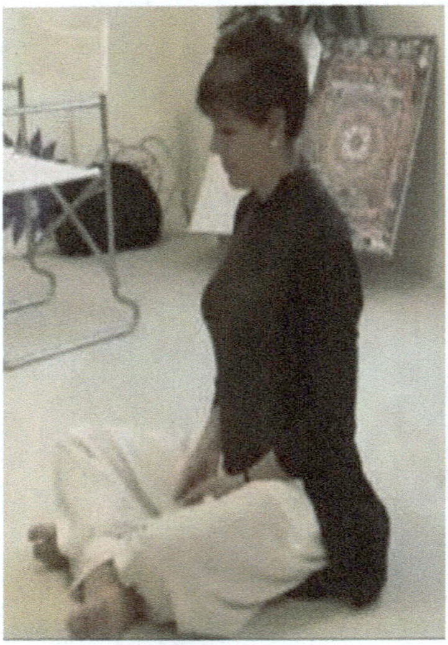

- Diamond posture: In this posture, you kneel with your buttocks supported on your heels. There are two versions. In the first one, a cushion is placed between your buttocks and the legs. In the second version, the pose is done without a cushion, although this can be uncomfortable when the meditation exceeds 15 minutes. In this case a special meditation box can be used that allows your buttocks to be supported without your weight falling on the heels. This posture is very stable and relatively comfortable.

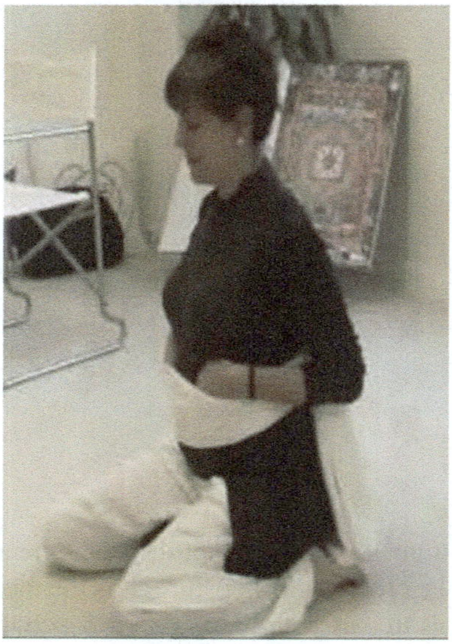

- Another possibility is to use an ergonomic chair specially made for meditation. This type of chair supports your buttocks and your knees in a stable and relatively comfortable position. The posture of your hands can be lying on your lap or, if necessary, you can wrap something around your waste to put your hands on.

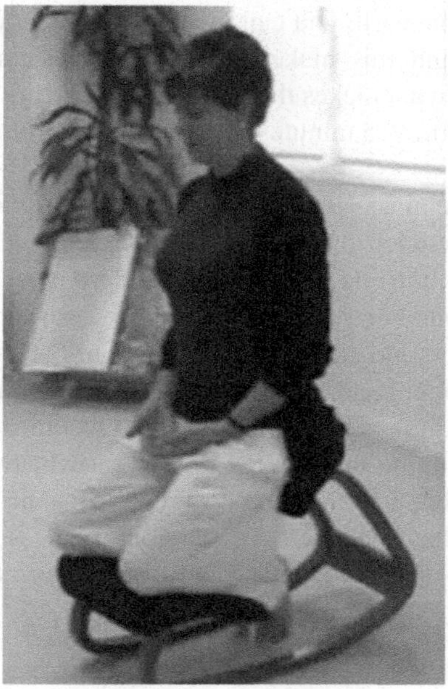

6 The Importance of Working into Compassion and Doing Homework

The Importance of Working into Compassion

Compassion-based interventions are relatively new, having only been established as a discipline in the past 20 years. As such, these types of interventions may still be relatively unknown and may run contrary to some of the basic assumptions in our society. This can make people resistant to compassion at times and therefore it is necessary to start the interventions slowly in order to work with the resistance appropriately.

It is also common for this type of intervention to generate a surge of emotions, so be careful to choose the amount and intensity of practice that works for you personally. You'll want to start with situations that are low levels of difficulty and work up to higher levels of difficulty that are moderately intense (between 6 and 7 on a scale of 0 to 10). In other words, don't use situations that are the most traumatic in your life.

Remember

It's better to start small and move forward as you feel ready!

Homework
Homework between modules (or chapters from this book) is a key part of the program. By doing the homework, you can incorporate the practices you learned into your day-to-day life, and this makes the benefits sustainable and long-lasting. Practice is a big part of what makes this intervention effective. About 20 minutes of formal practice and another 15 minutes of informal practice a day is usually enough to see a difference.

Enjoying the practice makes it that much easier to keep up.

Be careful! When it comes to doing or not doing the homework, we want to take the approach of compassion and not indulgence. Here is the difference:

Compassion seeks our long-term well-being in a sustained way, which is why daily practices are important because they change our habits.

Indulgence, on the other hand, seeks immediate gratification, even if it has a high personal cost in the medium and long term (e.g., it would be like a father who consents to his son not studying or allowing him to eat whatever he wants so that he does not get frustrated, but the long-term cost will be that he isn't educated or develops obesity). On the other hand, self-compassion practices are often rewarding on their own and produce some immediate relief from discomfort.

7 Informal Practice of 3 Compassionate Minutes

The Informal Practice, "3 Compassionate Minutes" will allow you to become aware of your environment, your body, your internal experience, and your breath, emphasizing the compassionate aspects of yourself and others.

This practice is one of the most important of the informal meditations and can be done at any time of the day. Plus, it's an easy way to start incorporating compassion into your everyday life.

And now, before finishing the module, let's practice… (Supplementary Audio 2.1).

You can find the instructions for the Informal Practice "3 Compassionate Minutes" in Annex 2.

Remember...

- Compassion can be understood as sensitivity to the suffering of others and a desire to help.
- When you direct compassion toward yourself, it's called self-compassion.
- Compassion can be used in different application contexts such as clinical, psychoeducational, and spiritual, which can vary in their objectives and forms of application.

- Attachment-based compassion therapy is based on (a) attachment theory, (b) contributions of religious/spiritual tradition, and (c) contributions of other models of compassion and other therapies.
- Formal practice involves selecting a specific place and time and using a specific practice or technique, while the informal practice does not have a specific time but is done at any time of the day (e.g., routine activities or time-outs).
- Working into compassion is key. It is better to start small and move forward as you feel ready.
- The Informal Practice "3 Compassionate Minutes" is a good opportunity to stop and become aware of your day to day, emphasizing the compassionate aspects with yourself and with other people.

8 Self-Assessment Questions

You're doing great! Now, let's review what you have learned in this module. For this, we will present you with a series of questions about the most important aspects. Don't worry if you don't know an answer; these questions are designed to help you.

Please answer the following questions:

	True	False
1. Self-compassion means being critical and harsh with yourself to overcome pain.	T	F
2. The most recommended meditation posture is lying on the floor.	T	F
3. It is better to meditate a little every day than to meditate sporadically for a long time.	T	F
4. The Informal Practice "3 Compassionate Minutes" aims to disconnect, distract you, and avoid the pain of others.	T	F

Explanation of Self-Assessment Questions

Question	Correct answer	Explanation
1. Self-compassion means being critical and harsh with yourself to overcome pain.	False	Completely false. To the contrary: self-compassion implies kindness and understanding of pain itself rather than being self-critical with yourself, perceiving your experiences as part of the human experience, and observing painful thoughts and feelings with perspective rather than over-identifying with them.
2. The most recommended meditation posture is lying on the floor.	False	The position of lying down on the floor, although it is usually one of the most comfortable, is only recommended in specific cases where the person cannot adopt other postures, since this position can make you sleepy.

Question	Correct answer	Explanation
3. It is better to meditate a little every day than to meditate sporadically for a long time.	True	Consistency is the key. Performing practices on a daily and regular basis produces greater benefits than intense and sporadic practices.
4. The Informal Practice "3 Compassionate Minutes" aims to disconnect, distract you, and avoid the pain of others.	False	Just the opposite! Informal Practice "3 Compassionate Minutes" will allow you to become aware of your environment, your body, your internal experience, and your breath, emphasizing the compassionate aspects of yourself.

9 Homework

Next, we are going to present you with a series of tasks. Carrying out the tasks that we propose in each module is a fundamental pillar of this program. The more you know and practice, the more you can benefit from the online intervention. Therefore, in addition to reading, listening, and reviewing all the information that is included in each module, we ask you to put the homework into practice. Think of a toolbox that you go to when you have a problem. We are giving you valuable tools. Now you have to learn how to use them. And don't forget: The more time you put into learning the material and doing the exercises, the more you'll benefit from it.

In this module we ask you to perform the following tasks:

- Read the content of this module carefully and review all the material included.
- Do Informal Practice "3 Compassionate Minutes" each day and try it at different times of the day, to see what works best for you.
- Experiment and practice different meditation postures to familiarize yourself with them or improve on them depending on your experience and physical abilities.
- Review the general advice on meditation and begin to create the conditions to establish the habit. Think about how to introduce meditation into your daily life, and if you already meditate daily, think about how to maintain and consolidate your practice.

Congratulations! You have finished Module 0 "Understanding Attachment-Based Compassion Therapy."

As you may have noticed, this is an introductory module. The goal was to introduce you to the program, explain what's involved, and how to get the most benefit from it.

Keep going! You're at the start of what we hope will be a rewarding journey of self-growth and discovery.

If you want, you can find the module summary in Annex 3.

Annexes of the Module 0

Annex 1: Attachment-Based Compassion Therapy for Self-Application

Modules	Theoretical content	Formal practices	Informal practices
0. Understanding Attachment-Based Compassion Therapy	What is Compassion Application contexts Attachment-Based Compassion Therapy: Explanation and Structure Use of Compassion in Meditation: Formal and Informal Practice General Tips on Practicing Meditation The Importance of Working into Compassion and Homework		3 Compassionate Minutes
1. Preparing for Compassion: Kind Attention	The Functioning of Our Brain The Reality of Pain: The Difference Between Pain and Suffering What Compassion Is Not	Compassionate Breathing and Compassionate Body Scan Compassionate Coping with Difficulties	Self Compassion Journal Gratitude
2. Discovering Our Compassionate World	Deepening the Concept of Compassion and Mindfulness Difference Between Compassion and Related Concepts Addressing Concerns About Compassion	The Figure of Affection Practice Develop a Safe Place or Situation The Compassionate Gesture and Compassionate Phrases Identify the Attachment Figure	The Object that Connects You to the World Compassionate Practice Journal What are You Good at?
3. Developing Our Compassionate World	Mechanisms of Action Through Which Compassion Works The Attachment Figure Effectiveness of Compassion Self-Criticism	Developing the Attachment Figure Substituting the Critical Voice for the Compassionate Voice	Letter from the Attachment Figure

Modules	Theoretical content	Formal practices	Informal practices
4. Understanding Our Relationship with Compassion	Biological Behind Compassion Attachment Patterns The Importance of Attachment Patterns in Daily Life Guilt Relationship with Caregivers	Practice to Identify Your Own Attachment Pattern Receiving Affection from Friends, Neutral People, and Enemies Repairing Guilt	Letter to Parents or Caregivers Observe How the Attachment Patterns Show Up in Daily Life
5. Working on Ourselves	Importance of Affection Toward Ourselves and Toward Others Shame	Give Affection to Friends and Neutral People Giving Ourselves Affection Repairing Shame Reconciling with Parental Figures	Greatest Show of Affection Ever Received Three Positive and Three Negative Things About Your Parental Figures
6. Understanding the Importance of Forgiveness	The Concept of Forgiveness Phases of Forgiveness Usefulness of Forgiveness Barriers to Forgiveness Resources to Use to Generate Forgiveness Recapitulation	Forgiving Yourself Asking Others for Forgiveness Forgive Others and Give Compassion to Enemies	Interdependence Compassion in Daily Life
7. Consolidating the Practice of Compassion	Work in Three Perspectives Usefulness of Being Your Own Attachment Figure Difficulties in Relationships Envy How to Maintain the Practice of Compassion Throughout Life	Become Our Own Attachment Figure Managing Emotions That Could Create Challenges in Relationships Working with Envy and Developing Joy for the Success of Others	Changing Your Perspective Our Values and Their Relation to Compassion Exercise 1 and Final Reflection: What Would Our Life Be Like if We Started Over?

Annex 2: Informal Practice: 3 Compassionate Minutes

Minute 1: Compassionately become aware of your environment, your body, and your inner experience.

Adopt the posture for meditation that you prefer and close your eyes. Then start to become aware first of the environment/place you are in (sounds, temperature, etc.) and of your body at the moment. Observe the contact of your legs with the mat or with the ground, the contact of your skin with the environment, or some pleasant or unpleasant sensation that you feel in your body at this moment. Channel a feeling of affection toward your environment: the earth that sustains you and the environment that embraces you. Now expand your awareness to all of your inner experience.

Spend a few moments asking yourself: What is your experience now? What thoughts are going through your head right now? What feelings or emotions are you experiencing? Are these feelings or emotions reflected somewhere in your body? Observe the sensations and emotions that appear at this moment, without judging them, showing affection and kindness to them, even if you don't like them.

Minute 2: Compassionate breathing

Direct your attention to your physical sensations and slowly bring attention to your breath. Slowly become aware of all the sensations of your breath at this time. Cradle your breath with affection, as if it were a small child. Don't try to modify it' just observe it in the present moment. If any thought or emotion comes up, let it go and return to your breath in a loving way, as often as you need.

Minute 3: Connection with humanity

Imagine that your consciousness looks like a transparent sphere inside your body that lovingly embraces you. Stay here imagining this for a few seconds. Now imagine this sphere, which is your consciousness, is progressively expanding, including all the people who are in this city. Feel united and identified with them. Stay with this feeling for a few seconds. Little by little, expand your consciousness to include this country and, progressively, to the entire planet. Feel united to all the people who live on our planet and to the entire cosmos. Remain with this feeling for a few seconds. And slowly, whenever you're ready, open your eyes.

Annex 3: Summary of the Module 0

Module Objectives

- Learn what compassion is.
- Understand the contexts in which compassion is applied and each of its objectives.
- Understand the theoretical bases for the intervention, including attachment theory and compassion meditation.
- Learn how to use meditation and learn the difference between formal and informal practice.
- Understand how to structure the practice of compassion meditation.
- Reflect on the importance of working into compassion and doing homework.
- Learn the Informal Practice "3 Compassionate Minutes" that will allow you to familiarize yourself with the concept of compassion in an approachable way.

Module Contents

What Is Compassion?

The concept of compassion in psychology is defined as "a sensitivity to suffering in self and others with a commitment to try to alleviate and prevent it" and when it is directed toward yourself it is called self-compassion.

What defines compassion is the desire to alleviate the suffering of another. Therefore, compassion is a motivation (and not an emotion) that guides human behavior.

Application Contexts

- Clinical level: The practice is aimed at patients who have a medical or psychiatric diagnosis and who want to treat or improve a specific illness (e.g., depression or anxiety).
- Psychoeducational level: The practice is aimed at people who do not have any clinical diagnosis and who seek to improve their general health and psychological well-being.
- Spiritual level: The practice is aimed at people (healthy or not) who pursue spiritual development and transcendence.

Attachment-Based Compassion Therapy: Explanation and Structure

The foundations of Attachment-Based Compassion Therapy are:

(a) Attachment theory
(b) Contributions from religious/spiritual tradition
(c) Contributions from other models of compassion and other therapies

It consists of eight modules with a duration of between 60 and 90 minutes each, and it is recommended to do one module a week, taking advantage of the time between modules to do homework.

Using Compassion Meditation: Formal and Informal Practice

The formal practice of meditation is done by selecting a specific place and time with a specific practice or technique, while the informal practice does not have a specific time but is done at any time of the day (e.g., routine activities or dead time like waiting in line).

General Advice on the Practice of Meditation

Where?: In a quiet place where you feel comfortable, with a pleasant temperature and dim lighting.

When?: Reserve a fixed time in your agenda to carry out formal practices, either as soon as you wake up, before going to bed, or at any other time of the day.

How much to meditate?: It is recommended to start for short periods of 5 to 10 minutes and gradually increase it over time.

How to meditate?: Adopting an attitude of openness and curiosity to the experience without expectations, as well as a comfortable posture that does not cause excessive discomfort or relaxation.

The Importance of Working into Compassion and Homework

Moving slowly and progressively into compassion is key. It is better to start small and advance as you feel ready. By doing the homework, you incorporate the practices learned in each module in your daily life with the aim to make the benefits sustainable and long-lasting.

Informal Practice "3 Compassionate Minutes"

This practice will allow you to become aware of your environment, your body, your internal experience, and your breath, emphasizing the compassionate aspects with yourself and with other people. This practice can be done every day, at any time of the day.

Homework

- Read the content of this module carefully and review all the material included.
- Do Informal Practice "3 Compassionate Minutes" each day, and try it at different times of the day, to see what works best for you.
- Experiment and practice different meditation postures to familiarize yourself with them or improve on them depending on your experience and physical abilities.
- Review the general advice on meditation and begin to create the conditions to establish the habit. Think about how to introduce meditation into your daily life, and if you already meditate daily, think about how to maintain and consolidate your practice.

Chapter 3
Module 1: Preparing for Compassion: Kind Attention

Module Objectives
In this module, we want to help you achieve the following goals:

- Understand the functioning of our brain.
- Learn and carry out the formal practices of compassionate breathing and the compassionate body scan.
- Reflect on the reality of pain: pain vs. suffering.
- Eliminate myths and inaccurate beliefs about compassion.
- Learn and carry out the formal practice of compassionate coping with difficulties.
- Learn and use the self-compassionate journal.
- Engage in gratitude exercises.

Go ahead with the module. Don't feel like you need to hurry through it. It's more important to try to understand all the concepts that are presented and practice the exercises.

Module Contents

1. The Functioning of Our Brain
2. Formal Practice 1: Compassionate Breathing and Compassionate Body Scan
3. The Reality of Pain
4. What Compassion Is Not
5. Formal Practice 2: Compassionate Coping with Difficulties
6. Informal Practice 1: Self-Compassion Journaling
7. Informal Practice 2: Gratitude
8. Self-Assessment Questions
9. Homework
10. Annexes

Supplementary Information The online version contains supplementary material available at https://doi.org/10.1007/978-3-031-38032-7_3.

J. García-Campayo et al., *The Attachment-Based Compassion Therapy*,
https://doi.org/10.1007/978-3-031-38032-7_3

In this module we will go over several concepts, including how our brain functions, the reality of pain in life, and what compassion is and isn't. In addition, we will introduce you to a series of practices, both formal and informal, to help you become familiar with the compassion in an approachable way. We also encourage you to use the self-compassion journal and do the gratitude exercise.

1 The Functioning of Our Brain: The Development of Our Brain Throughout Evolution

Most people want to be happy, and finding happiness is one of people's strongest desires. However, people were built for survival, and survival has historically been the main goal in life for humans.

All living things have the goal to eat and not be eaten by a predator (i.e., individual survival) and to reproduce (i.e., to survive as a species). Our body, and especially our brain, is specifically designed for this task.

However, a brain designed for survival doesn't fit with the goals of happiness and well-being. Our brains not only don't help us toward this goal of happiness, but may actually work against us.

Our brain *is not designed to be happy* but only to survive

For example, we tend to focus more on the negative things that happen to us than on the positive ones. This is because in the past negative situations threatened our survival.

We have a highly developed alert and threat system, which is easily activated. We can't freely deactivate this system, and it tends to continuously worry about the dangers. This is the source of much of our anxiety. Other animals only activate their alert system when they're in danger. And unlike us, they're able to deactivate it immediately as soon as they're safe.

The Evolutionary Structure of Our Brain

The structure of our brain developed over the course of evolution. Each evolutionary stage of the brain is associated with a different function, as shown in Table 3.1.

The more primitive brain (formed by the brain stem and limbic system) is also called the emotional brain. The more evolved part of the brain (formed by the neocortex) is called the rational brain.

Table 3.1 Characteristics of the three brains of humans

Brain	Structures	Functions
Reptilian	Brain stem	Defending territory, aggression and hunting behaviors, basic sexual behavior
Paleomammal	Limbic system	Caring for other group members, building alliances, engaging in play, attending to social rank and status, elaborate sexual behaviors
Neomammal	Neocortex	Ability to think about the past and future, think about own thoughts and emotions (metacognition) and what others will think of us (theory of mind)

Reference: MacLean, P.D. (1990). *The Triune Brain in Evolution*. Springer

Table 3.2 Positive (adaptive) and negative (maladaptive) aspects of the functioning of our mind

	Positive	Negative
Thinking about the future/imagination	+ Plan our life + Solve problems	– Create worry loops – Imagine terrible things
Thinking about the past	+ Learn from our past	– Brings up traumatic memories
Sense of self (i.e., who do we tell ourselves we are)	+ Integrate experiences	– Judge the way we act – Think about how other people will evaluate us

The original function of emotions was to move us to action. For example, anxiety might cause us to be alert and protect ourselves, and anger may cause us to defend ourselves from the threat.

The gap between the emotional brain (less developed) and the rational brain (highly developed) can make it difficult for us to adapt to our modern environment. This can also make it difficult for us to find happiness.

For example, thinking ahead helps us plan and problem solve, but we can also get caught up in worry loops and anticipating catastrophic events. Thinking about the past allows us to learn from our past but may also bring up traumatic memories.

In Table 3.2 below, we present the positive (adaptive) and negative (maladaptive) aspects about the way our mind functions.

The Attachment System

There is a specific brain circuit related to this intervention that we haven't discussed yet. It's called "The Attachment Circuit," and it's tied to our attachment system.

Mammals are the most social animals on the planet. Scientists believe that one of the main reasons for this is because mammals spend a lot of time caring for their young.

In fact, the children of mammals have the longest childhood: they are completely unprotected and at the mercy of predators for months and, in the case of humans, for several years. The cooperation of parents, and often other members of the group, is necessary to ensure survival.

This whole process of care and, specifically, the bond that is generated with the main caregivers is called "attachment."

Attachment is so important that there is a specific brain circuit for its maintenance that has been called "The Attachment Circuit." This circuit causes a newborn to observe a caregiver's eyes almost from birth or to smile within the first month of life, to reinforce protective behavior. Pregnant women also experience an increase in the levels of the hormone oxytocin which facilitates prosocial behaviors toward their offspring such as gazing, vocalizations, positive affect, and emotional contact. Therefore, as humans, we're predisposed to affection, care, and kindness.

During the first years of a child's life, the main caregivers provide the child with a feeling of protection, security, and affection, creating a "secure base." They give us a working model of how to deal with threats in adulthood.

However, if the child has not felt sufficiently loved and protected, his or her alert system becomes over-activated, which could make the person hypervigilant, and/or under-activated, which could make the person disengaged. This, in turn, could increase the chances of suffering or developing a psychological problem. Therefore, attachment is a key part of compassion.

2 Formal Practice 1: Compassionate Breathing and Compassionate Body Scan

Two formal practices are central to compassion interventions. They are "compassionate breathing" and "compassionate body scan."

Both practices are considered important to structure a new type of relationship with yourself, one that is more affectionate.

In addition, these formal practices can help you develop mindfulness. Mindfulness is a practice that we'll describe in more detail in future modules. It can help you quiet a wandering mind (focused on the present) and develop a compassionate attitude.

For this more affectionate relationship with yourself to become part of your life, we recommend regular practice of these two practices.

Here you will find the audios with guided meditations of "compassionate breathing" and "compassionate body scan," as well as instructions for each in annexes of this module.

You can do the two practices now or choose one of them and do the other at another time (Supplementary Audio 3.1 and 3.2).

3 The Reality of Suffering

The existence of suffering is one of the main ideas in compassion-based interventions. In other words, suffering is inevitable in life.

However, our modern world can make us think that suffering can be avoided and eliminated, which is not true.

The development of compassion is impossible without accepting the reality of suffering.

There is a difference between primary and secondary suffering:

- Primary suffering: Primary suffering as pain (or any unpleasant physical sensations you may experience) is inevitable, and we experience it because it is inherent to human nature, so we must accept it. However, accepting it doesn't mean resignation. It means accepting its reality without rejecting it. We may experience primary suffering (or pain) because of aging, illness, or death – either for ourselves or for our loved ones.
- Secondary suffering: Secondary suffering is avoidable. We create our own suffering when we don't accept the reality of pain (or primary suffering). Secondary suffering depends on what we tell ourselves and how we react to primary suffering.

An example of secondary suffering would be to lose a loved one (which is obviously going to cause us significant pain (or primary suffering) and think that no one will ever love us as much as this person. Or we might think that our life without that person will no longer make sense and that we will never be happy again. If we think these things, it's going to turn our pain (i.e., primary suffering) into secondary suffering.

Compassion helps us to reduce the secondary suffering. Some examples of this suffering are presented in Table 3.3.

Understanding the reality and universality of suffering is key to developing compassion, because the experience of pain is what makes all human beings equal

People who deny suffering, who do not accept it, or who do anything to avoid it, can't develop compassion for themselves or others.

One of the maxims of self-compassion is: "We do not give ourselves compassion to reduce suffering, but because we are suffering."

Table 3.3 Examples of secondary suffering

Fighting reality and not wanting to accept it	We are diagnosed with a serious illness, and we compulsively seek second opinions from other professionals, even in expensive hospitals in other countries, because we cannot accept the diagnosis
Feeling guilty or blaming others for events that are part of nature and life	After the death of a loved one, we blame ourselves for not having been there, or we blame other people for situations that are difficult to prevent (such as natural disasters) or that currently have no treatment (such as some diseases)
Anticipating the future	We suffer thinking that we can never be happy without a certain person in our lives, or we think that we will develop this or that disease in the future

4 What Compassion Is Not

1. Compassion is not pity

Hurt and grief are challenging emotions. We often become absorbed in our own problems when experiencing these emotions and forget that others have similar difficulties. Compassion assumes that we all experience suffering, and therefore, we don't need to feel pity for ourselves.

2. Compassion is not indulgence or looking for excuses

Compassion isn't about dropping everything and becoming passive. Rather, it's a genuine desire for health and well-being toward yourself and toward others. It's not about looking for indulgence in the short term (like the mother giving a child a chocolate bar so that the child doesn't cry), but instead it's about long-term well-being. In fact, people with high self-compassion are better able to stick to healthy habits like eating a healthy diet, exercising, or refraining from drug and alcohol use.

3. Compassion is not weakness

Many people believe that in a world as competitive as the one we live in, the practice of compassion will make them victims of predators. However, compassion is not at odds with assertiveness or standing up for our rights. It's a way of working with ourselves to reduce or prevent feelings of guilt, hostility, or envy and thereby increases our resilience and ability to cope with life's difficulties.

4. Compassion is not selfishness

The natural reaction when we're hurt or in pain is to take care of ourselves and recover. It's what any other animal would do because it facilitates survival. Loving ourselves in a situation of harm is not selfishness. In fact, when you take charge of your suffering and you take care of yourself, this enables you to be fully available to others. Self-compassion is a form of compassion, which is one of the most prosocial behaviors. In fact, self-compassionate people show more caring and empathy to others, which is why it is key in the helping professions.

5. Compassion does not diminish the motivation for change

You might think you need to be self-critical, or hard on yourself, to motivate yourself to change. However, self-compassion is far more effective for motivating change than self-criticism or self-punishment. Self-compassion can make it easier to see ourselves and our goals more clearly, as well as consider the costs of not changing and the benefits that will come from the new behavior. Self-compassion helps us recover from negative experiences and it's always easier to change when we're psychologically well.

5 Formal Practice 2: Compassionate Coping with Difficulties

When we have a problem and things go wrong for us, it's important to check what we say to ourselves.

Most of us criticize ourselves, we speak in a very harsh tone and even insult ourselves, and, in extreme cases, we blame ourselves and can be self-destructive.

The voice that appears in these circumstances is what we call our "self-critical voice," and the more frequent and intense it is, the easier it is for our discomfort to increase and our well-being to decrease.

This compassionate coping with difficulties exercise will help you identify your self-critical voice (Annex 3) (Supplementary Audio 3.3).

We also recommend doing this exercise informally in daily life, whenever you have a bad experience and say negative things to yourself.

You can adapt the things you say to yourself in the exercise based on what works for you. Practicing it will help you identify the words that are most helpful for you.

Table 3.4 describes the steps to be used in this practice.

Table 3.4 Steps to be used in the practice of compassionate coping with difficulties

Steps to be used in the practice of compassionate coping with difficulties
1. *Become aware of pain*: Acknowledge the experience and accept the pain you feel ("This hurts, I'm having a hard time.")
2. *Realize that pain is common* to all human beings (shared humanity). The particular difficulties and pain in general are part of a shared human experience of being alive ("Many people have experienced similar pain before, have this pain now, and will experience it in the future.")
3. *Recognize the impermanence* of all things: like any other experience in life, it will pass ("This will pass, like everything else in life.")
4. *Commitment to your self-care* (self-compassion): Instead of ignoring your own pain or punishing yourself, you want to love yourself and take care of yourself until the pain passes ("Right now, the best thing I can do is to take care of myself until all of this is over and I feel better.")

6 Informal Practice 1: Self-Compassion Journal

The self-compassion journal will help you reflect on how you talk to yourself, especially in stressful situations or when you are in pain.

We recommend that you structure this weekly diary into different sections (although you can do whatever works best for you). The following sections are typically included (Table 3.5):

In the Annex 4 you will find a template for a self-compassion journal. As you will see, in addition to completing the diary, we also recommend that you add a small final sentence with your self-compassion plans for the following week, whether you fulfill them or not.

Taking care of yourself and filling in the diary should not become an obligation that produces self-criticism, negative judgments, and more rumination. This would defeat the purpose of doing the diary. We can look for opportunities to love ourselves and take care of ourselves, but not make it an obligation where we critically evaluate ourselves.

Remember that the objective of doing this type of practice is to take care of yourself and love yourself as one of the basic activities in your life.

7 Informal Practice 2: Gratitude

Gratitude means to be thankful and feel appreciation. To have more gratitude in your life, try this simple exercise:

1. Identify 2 or 3 simple situations in daily life that bring you well-being or joy (e.g., being with friends having a drink, a sunset, playing with children or with a pet, a walk in the park, eating or drinking something that you like, etc.).

Table 3.5 Sections to structure the weekly self-compassion journal

Physical level	*What have you done to take care of your physical health?* Physical exercise, rest, diet, adequate sleep, periodic health check-ups, vacations, massages, etc.
Psychological-emotional level	*What have you done to take care of your emotional health?* Meditation, mind-body techniques, hobbies, spending time with pets, going on vacation, etc.
Friends-family relationship level	*What have you done to address your social life?* Spent time with friends, family, loved ones, wrote to them, restored old friendships, etc.
Values-spirituality level	*What are your values or meaning in life? What have you done in relation to your values?* Religious or spiritual beliefs, social or political commitment, environmentalism, nonprofit organizations, volunteering, etc.

2. Pause for a minute or two and savor these things slowly. By becoming more aware of the small pleasures in life, you can experience them more fully.
3. Express gratitude for life, for yourself, for others, and for being able to enjoy this moment.

The goal is to train your mind to not focus on only the negative or threatening aspects of life (negative emotions) but to identify and enjoy the positive situations and emotions even more.

Learning to have more gratitude is very important because emotions are self-perpetuating. If you only focus on negative experiences and emotions, you will continue to only notice the negative things. But if you learn to identify and enjoy positive experiences and emotions, you will start to notice them more and more.

Remember...

- Evolutionarily our brain is not developed for happiness, but for survival.
- There are three major evolutionary stages of our brain associated with different functions and characteristics. The gap between our primitive brain and our more evolved one can make it difficult for us to adapt to our modern environment and to find happiness.
- There is a difference between pain and suffering: a) Pain (or primary suffering): Inevitable and part of being human (e.g., aging, illness and death, both our own and those of our loved ones), b) (Secondary) Suffering: Preventable and created when we don't accept the reality of pain.
- Understanding the reality of suffering is essential to experience and develop compassion.
- Compassion will allow you to accept pain and will help you reduce suffering, by being more aware of your own pain and that of other human beings.
- Compassion is not pity, making excuses, weakness, selfishness, and it does not decrease the motivation for change.
- The bond that is created with main caregivers is called "attachment".
- Developing a secure attachment base is critical and is considered one of the goals of this intervention.

8 Self-Assessment Questions

You're doing great! Now, let's review what you've learned in this module. We'll present you with a series of questions about the most important aspects. Don't worry if you don't know an answer, these questions are designed to help you.

Please answer the following questions:

	True	False
1. Our brain pays more attention to positive situations than negative ones, which triggers our alert system, since in the past this was necessary for survival.	T	F
2. Compassion means pity or pity for others.	T	F
3. The attachment that we created with our caregivers serve as a model or guide for dealing with difficulties in adulthood.	T	F
4. The difference between pain and suffering is that pain is inevitable.	T	F

Explanation of Self-Assessment Questions

Question	Correct	Explanation
1. Our brain pays more attention to positive situations than negative ones, which triggers our alert system, since in the past this was necessary for survival.	False	Our brain pays much more attention to negative situations than to positive ones, and this triggers our alert system. This is to warn of danger because it was necessary for survival in the past. Evolutionarily our brain is not developed for happiness, but for survival.
2. Compassion means pity or pity for others.	False	Compassion means understanding that we all suffer equally, and not that we deserve special treatment from others. Pity is a negative emotion that tends to make the person become absorbed in their own problems and forget that others have similar difficulties.
3. The attachment that we created with our caregivers serve as a model or guide for dealing with difficulties in adulthood.	True	The bond created with our primary caregivers is called "attachment". In the first years of life, parents (or the main caregivers) provide the child with a sense of protection, security and affection, creating a "secure base". Such experiences with early caregivers help us develop a working model or guide on how to deal with threats in adulthood.
4. The difference between pain (primary suffering) and secondary suffering is that pain is inevitable.	True	Understanding the reality and universality of suffering is key to developing compassion, because the experience of pain is what makes all humans equal. Compassion will allow you to accept pain, and it will help you reduce suffering. Only by acknowledging suffering can we nurture and care for ourselves and others.

9 Homework

Next, we are going to present you with a series of tasks. As you already know, carrying out the tasks that we propose in each module is a fundamental pillar of this program. Remember, the more you know and practice, the more you can benefit from the online intervention. Therefore, in addition to reading, listening and reviewing all the information that is included in each module, we ask you to put the homework into practice. Think of a toolbox that you go to when you have a problem. We are giving you valuable tools. Now you have to learn how to use them. And don't forget: The more time you put into learning the material and doing the exercises, the more you'll benefit from it.

In this module, we ask you to perform the following tasks:

- Read the content of this module carefully and review all the material it includes.
- Do the formal practice of "compassionate breathing" and "the compassionate body scan" each at least once a week.
- Do the formal practice of "compassionate coping with difficulties" daily as well as when you experience a difficult moment or say negative things to yourself.
- Complete the "self-compassion journal" daily.
- In your daily life, identify two or three simple situations in which you are grateful (Informal Practice 2).
- Do any task/exercise/meditation we have recommended and you haven't done yet.

Congratulations!! You have completed Module 1 "Preparing for Compassion: Kind Attention."

You may have noticed that you're already becoming familiar with compassion. We encourage you to continue practicing everything you have seen in this module. You're doing great, keep going!

If you want, you can find the module summary in Annex 5.

You can also download the audio of the formal practices of this module.

Annexes of the Module 1

Annex 1: Compassionate Breathing

Adopt a comfortable position, with a straight back, but without effort, with your chest open and your eyes closed or semi-closed. Use a posture that's easy for you to maintain. Take one or two deeper breaths to bring attention to your body. Meanwhile, put both hands to your heart (or you can choose another compassionate gesture) to bring attention to the compassionate attitude that you will try to maintain during this practice. Little by little start to notice the sensations of your body in this moment (the contact of your body with the floor, with the mat or with the chair, the temperature of your skin, sensations in general, etc.).

Slowly, begin to become aware of your breathing. Pay attention to the movements of your chest and abdomen while you inhale and exhale or to the sensations of the air coming into and going out of your nose or mouth while you breathe. Feel affection toward your own breathing, toward your body, and toward yourself. You can express that affection by touching the area of your heart with one hand or hugging yourself. Keep in mind that the compassionate gesture you select should be comfortable enough to make it sustainable for a few minutes. You can lean toward your breath slightly as if it were a loved one, having the feeling that you take care of your breath, as if you were cradling it. It is important to follow the natural flow of your breath, without trying to change it, just observing it and becoming aware of it.

Your mind may wander due to some thought, feeling, or concern that arises. In these situations, you can be compassionate to yourself and simply become aware that your mind is wandering.

Kindly let distractions pass, without getting angry or judging them, and turn your attention back to your breath with the same gentleness that you would do with a little child who has been lost.

Feel how breathing nourishes your body, even if you are not aware of it. Feel gratitude toward your breath, toward your body, toward yourself, and toward the universe. Feel yourself merge with your breath, that you are your breath, and remain in that feeling for a few minutes.

Before closing the session, return your attention to the sensations of your whole body in this moment, and feel that everything is ok as it is, and appreciate the opportunity you have given yourself to take care of yourself doing this exercise. When you are ready, you can end the exercise.

Annex 2: Compassionate Body Scan

Adopt your usual sitting position for meditation, or, as is sometimes done when doing a body scan, you can lie on your back. Take a few attentive breaths, become aware of your body in general, and, if there is any area of tension, relax it.

Move your attention progressively to your head, your forehead (a place where we frequently hold tension), your eyes (take care that you don't press your eyes closed too much), your mouth (keep your tongue resting on the roof of your mouth, taking care that your lips don't press together too much), and your ears, and finally feel the inside of your head (brain). Perceive your whole face and head as a whole. If you notice pain or discomfort, pay compassionate attention to that part of your body, hoping that it recovers soon and thanking it for its role.

Move toward your neck and throat allowing them to relax and bringing your attention to any tension or discomfort. Continue down toward your shoulders. Bring your attention to both arms simultaneously, from your shoulders to your fingers passing through arm, elbow, forearm, and hands. Now go to your trunk, starting at your chest, filling your whole body with a feeling of goodness and affection. If you notice any discomfort, we invite you to soften and lessen it. Bring compassionate care to any pain or negative emotion. Do not resist it; let it be. If you are having problems in this period of life, let your hand rest on your heart, allowing this contact to comfort you and soften that negative emotion.

Continue with your abdomen and your stomach and then your sides and then your back and spine, subsequently feeling the internal core (heart, lungs, stomach and intestines, bladder, etc.). Bring compassionate care to any area of discomfort. You can also return to your breath or repeat the phrases: "I hope that I can be healthy," "That I can feel safe," "That I can have peace," or the phrases with which you most identify. You can simplify them by saying just one word: "peace," "health," "well-being," etc.

Next, bring your attention to both legs, from the top of your legs to the tip of your feet. If there are any tense areas, bring compassionate care to those parts. There may be times when it is very difficult to focus attention on some area of the body, because it is associated with an unpleasant memory. If so, you can skip that area if you prefer. Try to appreciate everything your body does for you.

End with a feeling of compassion for your whole body. Take notice of the areas of your body that you do not like, for aesthetic reasons (you don't like the look) or for functional reasons (it hurts). Try to appreciate your body as it is now, even though it's not perfect, because it allows you to be in the world, to kiss, hug, and relate. Progressively move the different parts of your body, and become aware of the room you're in. Try to carry this self-compassionate attitude toward your body for the rest of the day.

Annex 3: Compassionate Coping with Difficulties

Adopt the meditation posture that you usually use. Take several deep breaths to let go of any previous emotions and thoughts. Stay here a few moments, focusing your attention on the natural flow of your breath.

Little by little, begin to bring to mind a situation that happened in the last 6–12 months, when you experienced a problem, and you don't like the way you acted. Imagine the situation as completely as possible: remember what happened and what triggered the uncomfortable situation; it might be due to something someone said to you, a call you received, news you didn't expect, etc. Try to remember it as accurately as possible, as well as the way you reacted (what you said or did); it could be that you ran to tell what happened to a family member or a friend, or on the contrary, you kept it to yourself. Allow yourself to feel the emotion that you felt at that moment. When using mindfulness and compassion, we usually try to label and define the emotion that we're feeling. There can be several emotions tied together. For example, anger can lead to guilt, which in turn can lead to sadness. Remember what you said to yourself at that moment. You may have said words of criticism in a harsh tone.

We are going to replace that self-critical voice with a more loving one, and for this we will follow four steps:

First, recognize that you were experiencing pain (primary suffering) and that you were having a difficult time. There is no point in denying the pain because otherwise you will not be able to give yourself compassion. Recognize it by saying to yourself, "This hurt, I was having a bad time" (or another similar phrase). In this way, you become aware of your pain, so that you don't deny it, but don't stay trapped by it.

Second, realize that the experience of pain is common to all human beings by the very fact that we're alive. Recognize that the pain you experienced is part of what you can expect in life, but despite this, life is worth living. Recognize it by saying to yourself: "Many other people have experienced pain like this before, and, like me, others are experiencing it right now, and many more will experience it in the future."

Third, become aware that this pain, like all feelings and like everything that happens in life, is temporary. Recognize it by saying to yourself, "This will pass, like all things in life."

Fourth and the last step, try not to criticize or punish yourself, as you might do sometimes. Since you're experiencing pain and having a difficult time, you don't want to increase your pain even more, but stay committed to caring for and loving yourself until you return to feeling okay. If your pain is because you've made mistakes, there will be time to address the mistake when you're feeling better. But self-criticism does not help us to change; in fact it can make it more difficult to change. Recognize it by saying to yourself, "Look at how much pain (or suffering) I was in, let me take care of myself now to love myself while this pain lasts. I can make any changes I need to make when I feel better." When you say this, make the compassionate gesture that reassures you the most and stay as long as you'd like in this position, breathing calmly and giving yourself compassion. Finish by saying to yourself: "I hope I can come to accept myself as I am," or "I hope I can accept that it is human to make mistakes."

Annex 4: Template of Self-Compassion Journal

Self-Compassion Journal

Care areas	Monday	Tuesday	Wednesday	Thursday	Friday	Saturday	Sunday
Physical							
Psychological-emotional							
Friends-family relationships							
Values-spirituality							

Self-Care Plans for Next Week:

____

____

____

Annex 5: Summary of the Module 1

Preparing Ourselves for Compassion: Kind Attention

Module Objectives

- Understand the functioning of our brain.
- Learn and carry out the formal practices of "compassionate breathing" and the "compassionate body scan."
- Reflect on the reality of pain: pain vs. suffering.
- Eliminate myths and inaccurate beliefs about compassion.
- Learn and carry out the formal practice of "compassionate coping with difficulties."
- Learn and use the "self-compassionate journal."
- Engage in gratitude exercises.

Module Contents

The Functioning of Our Brain

The main goal of all species is survival. We are designed to survive, not to be happy.

We have a highly developed and useful alert and threat system from historic times when there were great predators. This system is easily activated, cannot be freely deactivated, and can result in continuous worrying and anxiety.

The Attachment System

The bond that is created with our main caregiver is called "attachment,"

In the first years of life, parents (or main caregivers) provide the child with a feeling of protection, security, and affection, creating a "secure base."

This provides a working model for how we deal with threats.

The Reality of Suffering: Primary Suffering (Pain) vs. Secondary Suffering

In life, there will inevitably suffering (i.e.,) pain as part of living and facing the situations that arise. Accepting the reality of suffering is key to developing compassion.

- Primary Suffering (Pain): It is inevitable and inherent to human nature (e.g., aging, illness, death of loved ones, etc.).
- Secondary Suffering: It is avoidable. We generate it by not accepting the reality of pain. It's what we tell ourselves and how we react to pain (primary suffering).

What Compassion Is Not

Compassion is not pity, making excuses, weakness, selfishness, and it does not decrease the motivation for change.

Homework

- Read the content of this module carefully and review all the material it includes.
- Do the formal practice of "compassionate breathing" and "the compassionate body scan" each at least once a week.
- Do the formal practice of "compassionate coping with difficulties" daily as well as when you experience a difficult moment or say negative things to yourself.
- Complete the "self-compassion journal" daily.
- In your daily life, identify two or three simple situations in which you are grateful (Informal Practice 2).
- Do any task/exercise/meditation we have recommended, and you haven't done yet.

Chapter 4
Module 2: Discovering Our Compassionate World

Module Objectives

- Deepen your understanding of the concept of compassion.
- Learn the main differences between compassion and related concepts.
- Understand the common concerns about compassion.
- Develop a safe place.
- Develop and practice the compassionate gesture.
- Start to identify the attachment figure.
- Practice and experience affection.
- Practice and experience compassion.

Go ahead with the module. Don't feel like you need to hurry through it. It's more important to try to understand all the concepts that are presented and practice the exercises.

Module Contents

1. Deepening the Concept of Compassion: Compassion and Mindfulness
2. Formal Practice 1: Connect with Basic Affection
3. Compassion and Related Terms
4. Formal Practice 2: Develop a Safe Place or Situation
5. Concerns About Compassion
6. Formal Practice 3: The Compassionate Gesture and Compassionate Phrases
7. Formal Practice 4: Identify the Attachment Figure
8. Exercise 1. What are You Good at?
9. Informal Practice 1: The Object That Connects You to the World
10. Informal Practice 2: Compassion Practice Journal
11. Self-Assessment Questions
12. Homework
13. Annexes

Supplementary Information The online version contains supplementary material available at https://doi.org/10.1007/978-3-031-38032-7_4.

J. García-Campayo et al., *The Attachment-Based Compassion Therapy*,
https://doi.org/10.1007/978-3-031-38032-7_4

In this module we will delve into the concept of compassion and its relationship with related concepts such as mindfulness. We'll also explore how it's different from other concepts, such as self-esteem. In addition, we will address concerns people can have about compassion.

We will ask you to do different formal and informal practices and exercises that will help you build the foundation of compassion.

1 Delving into the Concept of Compassion

Concept of Compassion from the Buddhist Perspective

The concept of compassion used in this intervention comes from Buddhism.

> One of the most frequently cited definitions of compassion comes from the Dalai Lama (2001): "Compassion consists of the desire for all sentient beings to be free from suffering."

In the Buddhist tradition, it's assumed that people automatically love themselves and find it difficult to love others. As such, Buddhism emphasizes loving others and having compassion for others.

This is encouraged in other traditions as well such as Christianity and Confucianism. In Christianity, we're told to "love your neighbor as yourself" and in Confucianism to "treat others as you would like to be treated."

However, you may experience the opposite problem, where you find it difficult to love yourself and easier to love others. This can then make it hard for us to have compassion toward ourselves.

Self-love, which has traditionally been viewed as the highest possible form of affection, seems to no longer be true in many societies because we having difficulty loving ourselves.

Qualities Required to Develop Compassion

According to Gilbert (2010, 2014), there are three qualities necessary to develop compassion.

- Mindfulness: To become aware of the suffering of others and of oneself.
- Strength: To be able to tolerate suffering without being trapped in it.
- Commitment: To try to reduce our own suffering and that of others to the extent possible.

The Importance of Practicing Mindfulness and Compassion Together

Mindfulness and compassion are sometimes described as "the two wings of the bird of wisdom." In other words, both mindfulness and compassion are essential to fly, so they are practiced together. They are complementary to each other.

To practice compassion, you also need mindfulness because you have to become aware of your own suffering and that of others, without judgment, attachment or rejection, to feel compassion toward the person who suffers.

In addition, practicing compassion requires a minimum level of attention that we can achieve with mindfulness.

To practice of mindfulness (e.g., breathing meditation or body scan) requires compassion so that we can have a kind attitude toward the experiences that arise in the present. Studies show that mindfulness interventions increase compassion. Although compassion is not specifically taught in most mindfulness exercises, implicit messages are included about the importance of being compassionate and kind to yourself and your mental processes.

When compassion and mindfulness are combined, it gives us the social commitment to try to make the world better and the individual commitment to love and care for ourselves when we are suffering.

In summary, compassion is a broad concept, and, in fact, studies suggest that it may be more effective than mindfulness for certain conditions such as depression (and other psychological concerns related to guilt and self-criticism) and for increasing psychological well-being in nonclinical populations.

Biological Differences and Specific Contributions of Compassion and Mindfulness

Biologically, there are big differences between the compassion and mindfulness. Mindfulness is a form of metacognition (being aware of one's own consciousness or cognition) and regulation of attention associated with the activity of the middle prefrontal regions of the brain, which is a more recent development in the evolution of the brain.

Compassion is linked to the mammalian care system and is evolutionarily much older. It involves oxytocin and other hormones related to the feeling of secure attachment as well as neural systems associated with love and affiliation.

The following Table 4.1 summarizes the specific contributions of each one.

As you might remember from Module 0, self-compassion is compassion directed toward the self.

Here's the paradox of self-compassion:

It involves both acceptance and change. It's only by accepting (and having compassion for) present pain that we can change (and reduce) future suffering.

Table 4.1 Specific contributions of mindfulness and compassion

	Mindfulness	Compassion
The question answered	What is your experience in the here and now, free from judgment?	What do you need right now to be well and reduce suffering?
Objective	Consciously focusing the mind in the present moment without judgment	Comfort in the face of suffering, Understanding that pain is an unavoidable part of being human
Risk of each component if not balanced with the other	Accept the discomfort of the person, forgetting their needs (affection), focusing exclusively on the experience. Eventual lack of motivation to reduce suffering	Not accepting the experience of pain (which is unavoidable). Not focusing on the here and now, or on the real nature of things, and wanting to find solutions for the future

To quote renowned psychologist, Carl Rogers (1995), "The curious paradox is that when I accept myself just as I am, then I can change."

2 Formal Practice 1: Connect with Basic Affection

The practice of connecting with basic affection (or practice of the figure of affection) is directly related to our affection and compassion for other beings (human or not). It's an essential step in compassion training and therefore cannot be skipped.

For some people, this practice can be simple and almost unnecessary, but for others it can be very complex.

The important thing, whether this exercise is simple or complex for you, is that you try it and continue practicing it. The ultimate goal of this exercise is that you identify a stable figure whom you can use to connect with the feeling of well-being, calm, and security at any time you want. This is especially important during times when you experience difficult emotions. You may need to do the practice several times before the figure of affection fully forms.

Keep in mind that many people have difficulties with affection. Before doing the practice, you can read some recommendations.

Recommendations When Developing the Figure of Affection and Connecting with Basic Affection

The figure of affection should be someone who is alive now. If the person has died, it's easy to feel grief and emotions associated with grief.

If it's a relative or someone very close to you, you may experience feelings of ambivalence toward the person if you also have conflict with them. This is common with parents, couples, and adult children.

It may be better to select someone or something with whom you have less of a relationship but also less conflict. A pet or someone else's small child can be a good choice as the figure of affection.

The figure of affection can be more than one person or animal. For example, people with more than one pet may feel guilty for including one but not the other. You can include two or three figures of affection.

Alright, now let's practice! (Supplementary Audio 4.1)

In the Annex 1 you will find the instructions of the Practice Formal 1 "The Figure of Affection."

This practice has a certain informative function. It is a kind of diagnosis of the ease or difficulty you have connecting with affection:

- If you find it very easy, this indicates that you have an easier time dealing with affection and compassion.
- If you find it difficult (or if you don't include people but animals or plants), this indicates that you have greater difficulty with affection and compassion or some distrust in people.

It is important to pay attention to this information as it can guide you on how to progress in the practice of compassion.

3 Compassion and Related Terms

Below you will find information about compassion and how it's different from related concepts.

Compassion and Loving-Kindness

Loving-kindness is a feeling of selfless love toward others (without attachment, without seeking personal gain) and reflects the desire that everyone be blissful and happy (Dalai Lama, 1997).

The main difference between loving-kindness and compassion lies in the absence or presence of suffering (primary and/or secondary).

- If there is no pain or suffering, the desire for others to be happy is "loving kindness."
- If there is pain and suffering, the desire for others to be free from it is "compassion."

In reality, loving-kindness is an aspect of compassion. Ultimately, it's all compassion since, by definition, there's always pain, even if sometimes it's not apparent.

Compassion and Empathy

Empathy refers to the ability to feel and understand the emotions of the other person. It is commonly described as "putting yourself in someone else's shoes." Empathy and compassion are not synonymous. This difference is evident in neuroimaging, because the brain areas involved in empathy are different from those involved in compassion. Empathy activates the brain areas involved in emotional aspects of pain, which makes sense because we can feel the pain of others. On the other hand, compassion activates the brain areas related to love and the desire to help others by relieving them of suffering.

Experiencing intense empathy for the person suffering can make us feel overwhelmed by the suffering of the other, which can lead to a negative experience. Compassion, on the other hand, produces positive emotions and feelings of affiliation, love, and care, which promote resilience.

Compassion and Emotional Contagion

Emotional contagion is when we experience the same emotions as another person, but in an involuntary way, and emotionally merge with that person, as if it was a "contagion." It usually occurs in people who have difficulty managing their emotions and who are easily influenced by others.

It is different from empathy, because empathy is voluntary and both people feel differentiated from each other. It is different from compassion, because with compassion we are aware of the other person's suffering, whereas emotional contagion involves fully merging with, rather than being aware of, the other person's emotions. By not recognizing the emotion of the other, it is not possible to evoke compassion or the desire to alleviate the other person's suffering.

Compassion and Sympathy

Sympathy refers to the emotion you feel for another person, specifically the feeling of concern for the other person. This positive feeling (or negative in the case of antipathy) is independent of whether you can understand the other person's feelings (empathy) or acknowledge their suffering and wish for their relief (compassion). However, empathy facilitates sympathy. In the same way, sympathy for a person could foster compassion, though compassion would be linked to the deep understanding of the reality of pain, that we all experience pain, and the desire to relieve it, beyond mere sympathy.

Table 4.2 Main differences between self-esteem and self-compassion

Self-esteem	Self-compassion
Answers to the question: Are you good enough? (compared to others)	Answers to the question: What do you need in order to be happy? (regardless of what other people think or want)
Based on global self-assessment: Needs to achieve goals in order to successfully compare yourself with others	Based on a kind relationship with yourself: Seeks to take care of yourself and give yourself affection when you are suffering
Looks for social comparison (what keeps us separate from others)	Seeks the connection with others (and brings us closer to them)
It depends on success: if there is no success, it can affect our self-esteem (and we can't always have success at something)	It doesn't depend on any other factor. It is always available, and we can use it with ourselves

Compassion and Altruism

Altruism is described as a helping behavior that benefits others, even though it could be harmful to oneself. Compassion focuses on the desire to alleviate suffering of another person but does not necessarily imply altruistic helpful behavior.

Compassion and Self-Esteem

Self-esteem is defined as the appreciation or consideration of oneself and is based on self-evaluation, in the search for personal success, and continuous social comparisons to check that we are not "below" others in the qualities that we are measuring. Compassion, on the other hand, places all people on the same level.

Without denying the usefulness of self-esteem, it has certain limitations in relation to compassion. In fact, self-compassion is associated with less negative affect and greater psychological health.

Compassion is related to the circuit of satisfaction, calm, and security, while self-esteem is related to the achievement circuit. Above all, it involves two very different ways of relating to ourselves. You will find the main ways in the following Table 4.2.

4 Formal Practice 2: Develop a Safe Place or Situation

Here's a common scenario: When we are young and afraid, often the best safe place is to be embraced by our mother or father (or main caregiver). When we are older, we experience situations of fear and insecurity at different levels, and, on many occasions, they can be difficult to face.

This practice involves developing a place (real or imaginary) where you feel safe and protected and where nothing bad can happen to you. It is also a place where you can feel calm and relaxed and where you can feel free to do whatever you want.

We encourage you to do this practice now (Supplementary Audio 4.2).

In the Annex 2, you will find the instructions of the Practice Formal 2 "develop a safe place or situation."

Over time, when you have developed your safe situation or safe place, the goal is to evoke it and experience that sensation whenever you want and especially after situations of insecurity, fear, or any other negative emotion.

This way you can activate the circuit of compassion to feel better.

5 Concerns About Compassion

Sometimes people reject using compassion because of concerns such as the following: (Kristen Neff, 2015, https://greatergood.berkeley.edu/article/item/the_five_myths_of_self_compassion).

- Compassion is a form of pity (i.e., feeling sorry for others or for yourself).
- Compassion indicates weakness.
- Compassion is narcissistic.
- Compassion is selfish.
- Compassion will make you complacent.

Research has found that these concerns aren't true. Specifically higher levels of self-compassion are associated with being more motivated to change problematic behaviors, being more psychologically adjusted, with engaging less in social comparison, to be more caring and supportive partners, and to have more secure attached relationships (Luberto et al., 2018).

People who struggle with perfectionism, self-criticism, guilt, or shame may have more concerns with using compassion, but may benefit from it the most (Kristen Neff, https://self-compassion.org/why-we-need-to-have-compassion-for-our-inner-critic/).

6 Formal Practice 3: Develop the Compassionate Gesture

Compassion interventions seek to regulate stress by activating the system of satisfaction, calm and security, linked to oxytocin.

There are certain gestures (related to hugging and contact) that release oxytocin, that is, they reassure.

The compassionate gesture can be very useful to reassure you in times of stress or just to feel better at any time.

We encourage you to experiment with different kinds of compassionate gestures and use the one that is the most effective for you.

Any of them can be carried out in private, but it is also useful to use one, less visible, in social situations that can be discreetly used in public.

On the other hand, the experience with the compassionate gesture can also help you convey better affection and security to other people.

And now ... let's practice! (Supplementary Audio 4.3)

In the Annex 3, you will find the instructions of the practice of the compassionate gesture.

Some of the most common compassionate gestures are summarized in the following Table 4.3.

In addition, the practice of the compassionate gesture can be accompanied by compassionate phrases. We encourage you to try it.

When a child is crying or when a friend is having a hard time, we try to calm them down by saying words that can help them cope with the negative emotion that they're experiencing. Along with the compassionate gesture, a key element in compassion is the use of compassionate phrases, which focus the attention and evoke the feeling of compassion/affection toward ourselves and/or toward others, which is the most healing element of the practice.

These phrases must be personalized and you need to develop them yourself, so that they're useful for you. The standard phrases developed by others, unless they serve you directly, tend to be less effective because they may not feel like they fit.

We recommend that the phrases meet a series of requirements:

- *Form of the Sentences*: We recommend that they're:
  - Brief, simple, and clear so that they reach you directly.

Table 4.3 Some examples of compassionate gestures

1.	Put a hand or both on your heart or in the central area of your chest. In both cases, your hands can remain fixed or caress that area (e.g., making circles or other slow movements)
2.	Put a hand on your heart or in the central area of your chest and another on your abdomen, in both cases your hands can remain fixed or caress
3.	Hugging yourself and caressing your arms
4.	Hugging yourself and caressing your back
5.	Put both hands crossed on your lower abdomen
6.	Cross your arms and caress yourself without actually hugging
7.	Patting yourself in the shoulder with one hand or both hands
8.	Caressing your legs (at different levels: thighs, legs)
9.	Cradle your face with both hands open
10.	Caressing the back of your hands, rubbing your hands, touching the fingertips of both of your hands
11.	Caressing your cheek
12.	Stroking the hair on your head
13.	Caressing your forehead

Note: The last ones from 10 to 13 are especially useful to do in public because they are very discreet

  - Sincere: if you don't believe what you say or it makes you feel bad in any way, you must modify the phrase until it doesn't cause you discomfort but a feeling of gratitude and well-being.
  - Kind, without judgments or criticism.
  - Not obligations (I have, I must).
  - Answers to the key question of compassion: What do I need now to be okay?
  - Consistent with the emotion.

- *Way of Expressing Them*
  - The diction must be slow; it is not a repetitive mantra, but rather you want to evoke feelings.
  - The tone used is whispering with affection, it must be as affectionate as possible, as if speaking to a child (we're really speaking to our inner child who is feeling insecure).
  - Don't use your official name (e.g., Robert) but the one that friends and loved ones use with you (e.g., Bob).

Usually it takes time to develop these phrases, and they may come about during different periods of mediation. It might take a while to decide the general structure of these phrases. Over time you can change them and modify some of the existing ones, etc. However, in general, if you feel them deeply you will tend to keep them for years.

We could say that, broadly speaking, there are two types of phrases depending on the scope of the needs that they cover: general and specific phrases.

General

They address the basic needs and expectations of the human being that equal us to all other living beings: the pursuit of happiness and the avoidance of suffering.

They are phrases of the type:

✓ "May I find happiness" (not specified in what concrete way).
✓ "May I be free from suffering."
✓ "May I find peace."
✓ "May my expectations and wishes be fulfilled."
✓ "May everything go well for me."

Specific

✓ "May I feel safe" (in cases of trauma, wars, etc.).
✓ "May I be healthy" (in cases of illness).
✓ "May I feel loved" (in cases of emotional breakdowns, conflicts with loved ones).

✓ "May I have peace" (in cases of family or work disputes or conflicts).
✓ "May I feel recognized" (in cases of work or family environments of continuous criticism).
✓ "May I come to accept myself as I am" (when there are aspects of myself that I do not like).
✓ "May I accept that it is human to make mistakes" (when I feel that I have made a mistake).

A key issue is that phrases have to express realistic wishes, not changes in the way of being of other people. Phrases of this type that do not depend on us do not make sense:

✗ "May (name of person) come to love me or forgive me."
✗ "May my son/daughter/child change his/her/their way of being."
✗ "May my parents love me."

7 Formal Practice 4: Identify the Attachment Figure

In life you will face adverse situations of all kinds and of different intensity levels which will test your ability to cope.

When we're children and face adverse situations, we'll often look to our parents or caregivers and wait for their reaction. We do this because our caregivers are our role models, and they give us a frame of reference for how to react.

As adults, it's also useful to have a figure of reference when things aren't going well for us: the attachment figure.

The attachment figure is someone who has all of the characteristics you consider essential to your security and well-being. This is someone who you see as stronger and wiser and whom you can turn to when you're not feeling safe or when you're suffering.

In Formal Practice 4, you'll identify whether or not this attachment figure exists and whether it's useful to you.

Try the following audio (Supplementary Audio 4.4)

In Annex 4, you will find the instructions for the Formal Practice 4 "Identify the Attachment Figure."

It may be necessary to do the practice several times with different adverse situations. The objective of this exercise is:

- To determine whether you usually use an attachment figure or not.
- If you do: we want to know what characteristics this figure has and if it's useful to you. If you don't use it, we want to know if you think it can be useful to you when you have problems.

If you have an attachment figure, it's important for you to know that you can enhance its effectiveness with practice. If you don't have such a figure, don't worry, it is possible to develop it so that it can serve you in difficult situations.

8 Exercise 1. What Are You Good At?

In the same way that our mind focuses on negative external stimuli, the same happens with the valuation of ourselves.

If we ask you, what are your weaknesses? Or what activities or knowledge are you bad at or are harder for you?

Chances are that the answer will come to you quickly and spontaneously.

On the other hand, if we ask you what activities, knowledge, or anything else you're good at, it's possible that you get stuck and don't know what to answer because you're not used to thinking and talking about your strengths. The goal is not to develop narcissistic pride but to make you aware of your strengths and consolidate them.

In this exercise we ask you to reflect on this. So, what are you good at?

We recommend that once you have reflected on what you are good at, you write it down somewhere so you can review from time to time (e.g., mobile notepad, notebook that you usually carry with you, post-it, etc.).

Try it out!

9 Informal Practice 1: The Object that Connects You to the World

This informal practice, which you can do as a homework task, consists of identifying a small portable object that you can carry in your pocket or bag, which you feel that connects you with the world.

It can be a memory of a person or living being to whom we have great affection (e.g., the photo of our children, a teacher, a pet, etc.), an object of great beauty that we feel connects us with the planet, or the photo of a masterpiece of humanity that connects us with the entire human species, etc.

You might take some time to identify it. The idea is that it's an object that you can always carry with you and that its mere presence makes you feel good, not because of a feeling of narcissistic self-esteem but because you feel that it connects you with humanity or with the planet.

10 Informal Practice 2: Compassion Practice Journal

The compassion practice journal is an important part of the intervention since it provides a record of what you practice, and it can help you observe your progress with meditation.

A quantitative diary can be made (like the example that you can download below) taking note of the type of practices that are done during the week, for example, as well as the time each technique is performed.

The weekly diary includes, on each day of the week, the number of times you meditated, at what time of the day (morning, afternoon, and night), as well as the total number of minutes you meditated. There is also a short line of observations in case you want to describe any relevant experiences that you have experienced.

Below, in the Annex 5, you can find a sample of compassion practice journal for your daily practice of compassion.

Remember

- One of the definitions of compassion from the Buddhist perspective refers to the wish for all beings be free from suffering.
- The practice of the "figure of affection" is aimed at connecting with feelings of basic affection to foster compassion.
- The three qualities or attributes necessary to develop compassion are mindfulness, strength, and commitment.
- Mindfulness and compassion are considered the two wings of the bird of wisdom, and it is thought that both are essential to fly, so they are practiced together. Therefore, they're considered complementary.
- Mindfulness is a form of metacognition (being aware of one's own consciousness or cognition) and regulation of attention, while compassion is linked to the system of care.
- There are several concepts related to, but different from, compassion such as empathy (feeling and understanding the emotions of another), emotional contagion (experiencing the emotions of another involuntarily), sympathy (positive emotion felt for another person), and altruism (behavior that benefits others even though it may be harmful to oneself).
- The formal practice of "develop a safe place or situation" consists of developing a (real or imaginary) place where you feel safe and protected, where nothing can happen to you.
- People who struggle with perfectionism, self-criticism, guilt, or shame may have more concerns with using compassion but may benefit from it the most.
- The "compassionate gesture" practice can be very useful to reassure you in times of stress or just to feel better at any time.

- The attachment figure refers to a reference figure, a role model, who can be useful when things are not going well.

11 Self-Assessment Questions

You're doing very well! Now, let's review what you have learned in this module. For this, we will present you with a series of questions about the most important aspects. Don't worry if you don't know an answer, these questions are designed to help you.

Please answer the following questions:

	True	False
1. The figure of affection can't be more than one person or animal.	T	F
2. To practice compassion you need mindfulness	T	F
3. The safe place aims to avoid or escape discomfort.	T	F

Explanation of Self-Assessment Questions

Question	Correct answer	Explanation
1. The figure of affection can't be more than one person or animal.	False	The figure of affection can refer to more than one living being. Therefore, two or three people or animals can be included in the same practice. This can occur in parents with more than one child or if they have more than one pet, since the person may feel guilty for including one and not the other.
2. To practice compassion you need mindfulness.	True	Right! To practice compassion, you need mindfulness because you have to become aware of your own suffering and that of others, without judgment, attachment or rejection, to feel compassion toward the person who suffers.
3. The safe place aims to avoid or escape discomfort.	False	This practice consists of developing a place (real or imaginary) where you feel safe and protected and where nothing bad can happen to you. It is also a place where you can feel calm and relaxed and where you can feel free to do whatever you want. The safe place allows you to face situations of insecurity, fear, or some other negative emotion. In the long term, the goal is for you to evoke this safe place and experience the sensation(s) it brings up whenever you need to.

12 Homework

Next, we are going to present you with a series of tasks. As you already know, carrying out the tasks that we propose in each module is a fundamental pillar of this program. Remember, the more you know and practice, the more you can benefit from the online intervention. Therefore, in addition to reading, listening and reviewing all the information that is included in each module, we ask you to put the homework into practice. Think of a toolbox that you go to when you have a problem. We are giving you valuable tools. Now you have to learn how to use them. And don't forget: The more time you put into learning the material and doing the exercises, the more you'll benefit from it.

In this module we ask you to perform the following tasks:

- Read the content of this module carefully, and review all the material it includes.
- Do Formal Practice 1 "Connecting with Basic Affection" at the least once. Depending on your situation, we recommend doing the practice several times a week on alternate days.
- Do Formal Practice 2 "Develop a Safe Place or Situation" at least once. Depending on your situation, we recommend doing the practice several times a week on alternate days.
- Do Formal Practice 3 "Compassionate Gesture" at least once, and try to identify the compassionate gesture that's most effective for you.
- Do Formal Practice 4 "Identify the Attachment Figure" to the least once.
- Evoke the figure of affection several times a day to feel better and whenever you feel bad (or not loved).
- Remember the safe place when you feel uneasy.
- Use the compassionate gesture daily (and compassionate phrases, if you'd like).
- Do Exercise 1 "What Are You Good at?"
- Do Informal Practice 1 "The Object that Connects You to the World."
- Use the "compassion practice journal" to record your meditative practice daily.
- Keep practicing the formal practice of "compassionate breathing" and "compassionate body scan" at least once a week each.
- Review any previous module that you have questions about.
- Do any task/exercise/meditation that we have recommended and you haven't done yet.

Congratulations!! You have completed Module 2 "Discovering Our Compassionate World."

In this module you have delved into the concept of compassion and its relationship with other concepts, advancing the practice of compassion.

We encourage you to continue practicing everything you have seen in this module. Keep going, you're building your compassion skills that will continue to benefit you in your everyday life.

If you want, you can find the module summary in Annex 6. You can also download the audio of the formal practices of this module.

Annexes of the Module 2

Annex 1: Formal Practice 1 "Practice of the Figure of Affection"

Adopt the meditation posture that you usually use. Observe for a few moments how your body feels and any sensations you have. Take several deep breaths, with attention, to be able to let go of previous emotions and thoughts. Little by little, begin to bring to mind the image of some living being that makes you feel good, produces tenderness, or simply makes you smile or relax. This image may be that of a loved one, of an animal (e.g., pet), or a plant (e.g., flower).

The idea is to evoke something or someone that is alive at this moment and that helps you feel well-being, peace, love, etc. Stay a few seconds choosing that figure. It is important that the figure you choose does not generate any conflicting feelings, and for this reason, we recommend not to think about a partner, parents, or an adult child, with whom it is common to have contradictory feelings.

If during practice you observe that no figure appears spontaneously, if nothing happens, you don't have to force it. You are exploring this topic. It will develop over time. If it appears, observe what characteristics the figure has, how it makes you feel, and why you have chosen it. Stay a few seconds with that feeling.

Little by little, let go of any visualization or mental images that may have appeared during the practice. And when you're ready, you can open your eyes, move the different parts of your body, and return your attention to the room you're in.

Annex 2: Formal Practice 2 "Develop a Safe Place or Situation"

The practice can be done sitting or, better yet, lying down, with the possibility to adopt a fetal position. Choose the position in which you're most comfortable.

Stay for a few moments noticing how your body feels and the sensations that arise. You may be relaxed and calm or perhaps anxious and fatigued. Accept the experience as it arises, without judging it. Little by little, turn your attention to your breath, to let the emotions and thoughts that arise pass through, and stay in this process for a few moments. No matter how many thoughts appear or the content they have, let them pass without fighting them, without rejecting them, or getting attached.

Now, imagine a situation or a place (real or imaginary) in which you feel that nothing bad can happen to you, in which you feel absolutely safe. This place may be known to you, for example, somewhere you used to go when you were little, a house that made you feel protected and safe, a landscape that you like and transmits you serenity, etc. You can modify it or recreate it in your mind as it is. If you prefer or find it easier, it can be completely imaginary, and you can decorate it at will. Look at the characteristics of this place: what shape it has, what furniture or objects are there, what color predominates, what characteristics it has, what are you doing when you are in this place, whom do you meet, etc. It's important that the place is what brings the feeling of security, and not the presence of someone else in the space. You can use or create any place or situation that works for you.

When you do the practice several times, the image will stabilize and become enriched with new details. The important thing is the feeling: You have to be able to feel absolutely calm and at peace, with the certainty that nothing bad can happen to you, a place where you feel free and you can do whatever you want, even if it's impossible (e.g., flying). You might get the sense that the place itself is glad that you feel calm and happy there. You can think about why you like to be in this place and what it is that makes it safe for you.

Little by little, when you're ready, open your eyes, move the different parts of your body, and return to the room you're in, ending the practice.

Annex 3: Compassionate Gesture Practice

Begin by adopting the meditation position that you usually use, and spend a few moments observing the sensations that arise in your body. Now, take several deep breaths, very slowly and with attention, in order to let emotions and previous thoughts pass through you. Breathe in and out, feeling how your body fills with energy with each inhalation and how it relaxes and frees itself from resistances with each exhalation.

Now, we will have you make a series of compassionate gestures, being aware of the sensations and emotions that arise.

The most classic gesture is hugging. Keeping your eyes closed, do this now and hug yourself. Caress your arms and back and observe the sensations that appear. The hug gesture is usually very powerful, since it triggers oxytocin, producing a feeling of well-being. Stay in this compassionate gesture of embracing yourself for a moment.

You can now try to put your hands on your heart. You can feel your heart beat and the life in your body. You can place one hand on the heart and the other on the abdomen or even both hands on the chest, or on the heart; you are trying out and trying to identify with which of all the gestures you feel most comfortable.

You can now caress your legs; many people do it when they are nervous or restless, but it can be a gesture of affection as well. Stay a few moments feeling the sensations that appear.

Now turn, with full attention, to gestures associated with your face. Try sliding your hand down your cheek, or place it on the top of your head. The smooth movement of the hand across the head can give a feeling of considerable calm.

You can also try to caress your hands and touch the tips of your fingers together.

It's often helpful to perform this practice more than once, to decide which are the best compassionate gestures for you. Whenever you have a feeling of discomfort or sadness, you can make the compassionate gesture you choose that connects you with the feeling of security. Physical contact is very healthy, both with children and with family members or with yourself. Try to use it as much as you can in daily life.

Now, little by little, begin to move slowly, and open your eyes, ending the practice.

Annex 4: Formal Practice 4 "Identify the Attachment Figure"

Practice of Identifying the Attachment Figure

Adopt the meditation position that you usually use. Take several deep breaths, with attention, to let previous thoughts and emotions pass.

Bring to your mind some recent situation (in the last 6–12 months) in which you felt bad. To begin, we recommend not choosing the most traumatic situation of your life but one of mild/moderate intensity.

Start by developing the scene: Remember what you were doing, who you were with, what you and the others said, and what happened. Connect with the emotion you feel remembering this, and identify it (you may be feeling several different emotions). Try to name the emotion: anger, sadness, fear, etc.

Remember what you were thinking, what you were feeling at the time, and how you acted. Try to remember if at any moment you thought about how a person who is important to you, someone who serves as reference, would react or what would they say about the situation. If you think of a person or figure of this type, analyze who it was and what characteristics they had, and why they were important to you. If you didn't think about such a figure, reflect about whether it would be useful to have such a figure when you face adverse situations, and why.

Annex 5: Example of Compassion Practice Journal

	Monday	Tuesday	Wednesday	Thursday	Friday	Saturday	Sunday
Number of times							
Total minutes							
Day period (M, A, N)							
Observations[a]							

Note: *M* morning, *A* afternoon, *N* night
[a]You can specify the type of compassion practice you have done, as well as any other aspects or observations you have experienced during the practice

Annex 6: Summary of the Module 2

Objectives

- Deepen your understanding of the concept of compassion.
- Learn the main differences between compassion and related concepts.
- Understand the common concerns about compassion.
- Develop a safe place.
- Develop and practice the compassionate gesture.
- Start to identify the attachment figure.
- Practice and experience affection.
- Practice and experience compassion.

Deepening the Concept of Compassion

Compassion consists of the wish that all sentient beings be free from suffering. Mindfulness and compassion are considered the two wings of the bird of wisdom. To practice compassion, minimum levels of attention are necessary, which are practiced with mindfulness, and mindfulness interventions increase compassion.

There are three qualities to develop compassion:

- Mindfulness (or full attention)
- Strength
- Commitment

Biological Differences and Specific Contributions

Mindfulness is a form of metacognition and attention regulation, making it a recent evolutionary achievement. On the other hand, compassion is linked to the care system and is evolutionarily older. Compassion is related to secure attachment, love, and affiliation.

Specific Contributions

- Mindfulness answers the question: What is the experience here and now?; compassion answers: What do you need now to be well and reduce suffering?
- Regarding objectives: Mindfulness helps to become aware of the experience of the present and accept its nature. Compassion comforts in the face of suffering.
- The risk of each intervention if not balanced with the other:
  - In Mindfulness: accept the discomfort forgetting the needs.
  - In Compassion: not accepting the experience of suffering.

Compassion and Related Terms

Loving-kindness refers to a feeling of selfless love toward others (without attachment, without seeking personal gain) and reflects the desire that everyone be blissful and happy (Dalai Lama, 1997).

If there is no suffering, the desire for others to be happy is "loving-kindness"; if there is suffering, the desire that others be free from it is "compassion."

Concerns About Compassion

Sometimes, it can be thought that the one who gives compassion would have a certain moral superiority over the one who receives it. Some may think that compassion indicates weakness. However, compassion occurs among equals and is independent of being assertive or standing up for our rights.

Homework

- Read the content of this module carefully and review all the material it includes.
- Do Formal Practice 1 "Connecting with Basic Affection" at the least once.**
- Do Formal Practice 2 "Safe Place" at least once.**
- Do Formal Practice 3 "Compassionate Gesture" at least once and try to identify the compassionate gesture that's most effective for you.
- Do Formal Practice 4 "Attachment Figure" to the least once.
- Evoke the figure of affection several times a day to feel better and whenever you feel bad (or not loved).
- Remember the safe place when you feel uneasy.
- Use the compassionate gesture daily (and compassionate phrases, if you'd like).
- Do Exercise 1 "What are You Good at?"
- Do Informal Practice 1 "The Object that Connects You to the World."
- Use the "compassion practice journal" to record your meditative practice daily.
- Keep practicing the formal practice of "compassionate breathing" and "compassionate body scan" at least once a week each.
- Review any previous module that you have questions about.
- Do any task/exercise/meditation that we have recommended and you haven't done yet.

** Depending on your possibilities, it is recommended to do the practice several times a week on alternate days.

Chapter 5
Module 3: Developing Our Compassionate World

Module Objectives
In this module, we want to help you achieve the following goals:

- Understand the mechanisms of action through which compassion works.
- Develop your own attachment figure, which is one of the core elements of compassion.
- Learn the types of disorders that compassion can be effective for.
- Learn what self-criticism is, the purpose it serves, as well as how to replace it with self-compassion.

Go ahead with the module. Don't feel like you need to hurry through it. It's more important to try to understand all the concepts that are presented and practice the exercises.

Module Content
1. How Compassion Works
2. The Attachment Figure
3. Formal Practice 1: Developing the Secure Attachment Figure
4. Effectiveness of Compassion
5. Self-Criticism
6. Formal Practice 2: Developing the Compassionate Voice
7. Informal Practice 1: Letter to the Attachment Figure
8. Self-assessment Questions
9. Homework
10. Annexes

Supplementary Information The online version contains supplementary material available at https://doi.org/10.1007/978-3-031-38032-7_5.

J. García-Campayo et al., *The Attachment-Based Compassion Therapy*,
https://doi.org/10.1007/978-3-031-38032-7_5

In this module we'll describe the ways through which compassion works and the types of psychological problems it's effective for. This information is intended to increase your motivation to get involved in the practice and increase the effectiveness of the intervention for you. We'll also explore the role of the attachment figure as well as the elements of self-criticism.

1 How Compassion Works: Mechanisms of Action

The compassion-based interventions (CBI) are still quite new, and we do not have definitive studies yet on the mechanisms of action (i.e., the way it works), although there are several hypotheses with some research to support them. Mindfulness is often a component of compassion; therefore we'll also consider the mechanisms of action specific to mindfulness.

Mechanisms of Action for Compassion

There are two types of action mechanisms, those specific to compassion therapy and those related to mindfulness.

Specific Mechanisms of Compassion

We're going to introduce you to the four specific mechanisms of action of compassion:

The first is *decreasing self-criticism.*

When self-compassionate people describe their weaknesses, they often don't feel as isolated or guilty. They might think about their weakness not as something only about them but as something that other people experience as well. For example, they might not use the first person singular ("I") but rather using the plural ("we") and making more social references (to family, friends, and others human beings), due to the greater connection and kindness with themselves and with other people.

The second mechanism is *decreasing rumination*. People with more self-compassion have less rumination. That is, they remain less hooked by thoughts about the past and accept their own imperfections with greater self-compassion. This decrease in rumination is an explanation for why higher self-compassion is associated with lower occurrence of anxiety and depression (e.g., Krieger et al., 2013; Wu et al., 2019).

The third is *developing a new interpretation of negative events*. Self-compassion allows us to see problems with more perspective, understanding that our problems are similar to those of most people.

And finally, the fourth mechanism is *regulating emotions*. Self-compassion makes it easier to cope with unwanted emotions and thoughts, because we recognize that our own emotions are valid and important.

Mechanisms of Action for Mindfulness, Specifically Related to Compassion

You just learned about the specific mechanisms of action for compassion. Now we are going to review the mechanisms of action for mindfulness that are related to the development of compassion. Therefore, we won't talk about all the mechanisms of action of *mindfulness* but only about those that could be related to the development of compassion.

Mindfulness works by increasing open and curious nonreactive attention to all stimuli (including those related to the suffering of others) and reducing affective bias. In other words, *mindfulness* increases psychological flexibility and openness when facing external situations and when regulating emotions.

2 The Attachment Figure

The attachment figure is the core element of compassion. According to attachment theory, individuals who, during childhood, grow up in unsafe or threatening environments and who experience constant criticism and aggression tend to be very self-critical and not very self-compassionate.

The aim of compassion techniques is to improve the relationship that we establish with ourselves, developing a secure attachment figure. To achieve this, compassion is trained through exercises of imagination, where we create and work with a compassionate image.

3 Formal Practice 1: Developing the Secure Attachment Figure

During the practice, you are asked to create or imagine your ideal compassionate figure. This is useful because it allows you to understand what makes a figure compassionate for you: Protection? Validation of your feelings? Understanding? Care?

These could be characteristics associated with a secure attachment figure. We want these characteristics that we associate to well-being, understanding, affection, wisdom, and any other positive aspect that is relevant to us.

And now, let's practice (Supplementary Audio 5.1).

In Annex 1 of this module, you will find the instructions of the Formal Practice 1 "Developmental Practice of the Attachment Figure."

It is very common for difficulties to arise when developing the attachment figure, and it will often be necessary for you to practice this exercise several times. Consider the following aspects that we point out:

- People with religious beliefs can sometimes develop an attachment figure based on representations of divinity or religious figures of protection.
- Those who do not have these beliefs often use important people in their life that have offered affection and wisdom, like teachers, family, or famous people for some characteristic associated with compassion (e.g., Dalai Lama, Mother Teresa of Calcutta, etc.)
- Parents can be used as attachment figures, although they are not usually recommended, since they often tend to be associated with ambivalent or negative feelings, and not only with positive feelings.
- Although some of these figures constitute the foundation of the attachment figure, we recommend personalizing the figure's characteristics, according to your own expectations about what compassion should be.
- For many people visualization is difficult, but the most important thing is the general feeling, as you want the figure to evoke a bond of security and compassion.
- It's common that at the beginning of the practice, you may not feel that the attachment figure has the qualities described. That's ok; the important thing is the intention that you want to develop the figure with those qualities.
- Once you have developed the attachment figure, it doesn't have to be final version, but it can be modified according to your preferences. You may also come to have more than one attachment figure.
- Often, over time, you may end up becoming your own attachment figure.

4 Effectiveness of Compassion

Efficacy of Compassion Therapy

Next, we're going to review the efficacy of compassion interventions for different diagnoses. Specifically, we'll present its effect on psychiatric and medical diagnoses (clinical level) and in individuals without diagnoses (psychoeducational level) but where compassion can be used to increase psychological well-being.

Effect on Different Diagnoses and Disorders

There are few meta-analyses (i.e., the studies that review clinical trials and compile all of the scientific evidence) on the efficacy of compassion-based interventions in different mental health conditions (Kirby et al., 2017; Austin et al., 2021; Wakelin et al., 2022).

In general, self-compassion is considered more effective than mindfulness in the treatment of depression. In anxiety disorders it is not so clear which of the two therapies is more effective, and it seems that it depends on the characteristics of the person. What is evident is that both interventions do not produce exactly the same results, and their combination is more beneficial than using either of them in isolation (Kirby et al., 2017; Austin et al., 2021; Wakelin et al., 2022).

Compassion appears to be especially helpful for conditions related to stress, social anxiety, and conflict in interpersonal relationships (e.g., relationship conflicts, caregiver syndrome) and all conditions that are associated with anger. In the following Table 5.1, we summarize other disorders in which compassion therapy has proven helpful.

Effect in Healthy People on Psychological Well-Being

Studies suggest that compassion could have a greater effect than mindfulness on satisfaction with life, happiness, and psychological well-being (Campos et al., 2016; Zessin et al., 2015). This does not mean that compassion is more effective than mindfulness but simply that they have different effects.

Self-compassion is associated with different psychological strengths such as greater emotional intelligence, wisdom, satisfaction with life, and feelings of social connection, all of which are important elements for the development of a meaningful life. Self-compassionate people also display more optimism, curiosity, creativity, and other positive emotions such as enthusiasm and inspiration, compared to more self-critical individuals. It should be noted that compassion's way of being effective is not by replacing negative thoughts and emotions with positive ones but by embracing and accepting negative thoughts and emotions as part of human nature (García-Campayo, 2019).

Furthermore, self-compassion is linked to more personal initiative, high efficacy, and intrinsic motivation. It is also associated with a greater ability to make changes that lead to self-improvement, learning from experience and avoiding previous mistakes. All these features make self-compassion very effective for the development of healthy behaviors that are linked to a strong motivation, for example, the maintenance of weight loss diets, the adherence to drug treatment, or physical exercise regularly (Phillips & Hine, 2021).

Table 5.1 Other conditions for which compassion therapy has been shown effective

Chronic pain	It reduces catastrophizing (and the perceived injustice) associated with this disorder
Eating behavior disorders	Including self-compassion in the early treatment of eating disorders seems to improve prognosis, since self-criticism seems to be one of the key elements in the worsening of the disease
Child psychological trauma	High levels of self-compassion achieve better emotional regulation in people who've experienced trauma, decreasing the impact of trauma, allowing them to cope with adverse events in a more effective way

5 Self-Criticism

Self-criticism is defined as the criticism that an individual makes of themselves. In psychology we refer to that internal ruminative dialogue that may resemble depression. Self-criticism usually appears in the early years of childhood, generally caused by caregivers (especially demanding and critical caregivers).

In principle, self-criticism is often meant to help us achieve certain things that aren't necessarily negative, since they were established by our parents or teachers who, in most cases, wanted the best for us (although their perspective might seem wrong to us).

Studies confirm that the problem is not so much the content of the criticism (e.g., do this or do that; you have to be or get this or that) but the tone and negative emotions associated with that criticism. There are two main types of self-criticism:

- Criticism related to feeling inferior and like a disappointment: It appears in the general population and is the most common type of criticism. This is often the result of having parents or teachers who systematically use destructive criticism with an emotional tone of disappointment.
- Criticism related to self-hatred: This is less common and usually appears in populations with psychological conditions. Often if there's been some type of child abuse.

The Goal of Self-Criticism

Self-criticism is when we evaluate our own behavior and attributes, which often involves judging ourselves for our own weaknesses, errors, and shortcomings. Although, self-criticism can have a positive effect in fostering personal growth, a tendency toward harsh self-criticism is thought by some to be a risk factor for depression (American Psychological Association, https://dictionary.apa.org/self-criticism).

We can say that self-criticism has two main objectives:

1. *Warning*: It causes us to pay attention to something that makes us afraid, something that could have terrible consequences if we're not careful (e.g., if you do not do everything that people ask you to do, no one will love you).
2. *Sense of control*: There's much in life that we don't have control over (where we were born, when we will get sick or die, when our loved ones will die, etc.). Self-criticism gives us a sense of control over life events. For example, if we failed an exam or aren't selected for a job, thinking that we haven't prepared enough for the exam or the interview may be true. But it also discounts the many factors that may have led to that outcome and were outside of our control. Self-criticism allows us to deceive ourselves that we can control our future by criticizing ourselves.

Self-criticism serves a survival function in situations of mistreatment or abuse. When damage is caused by "someone powerful" (parents, seniors, educators), the child's survival system is activated to prevent damage. Abusers are often unpredictable and cannot be changed; therefore the child's own behavior is the only source of alleged control. In this way, the child becomes hypervigilant to avoid behaviors that trigger the abuse. This can cause children to automatically blame or criticize themselves whenever they engage in any behavior that results in abuse. However, the abuse is not actually dependent on the child's behavior. The levels of abuse could have been very subtle, or the self-criticism could have been activated simply to not disappoint parents with high expectations of their children.

How to Replace Destructive (Self) Criticism with Constructive Thoughts

We all make mistakes, and we all have room for improvement. This applies to us as well as those around us.

For criticism to be effective and fulfill its objective (which is to motivate change and improvement, not to humiliate), it must meet a series of characteristics.

In the following Table 5.2, we summarize the differences between constructive and destructive criticism.

As the diagram below indicates (Fig. 5.1.), criticism can be constructive or destructive, and it can be focused on the self or on others. In the next section, we focus specifically on destructive self-criticism.

Table 5.2 Differences between constructive and destructive criticism

Constructive criticism	Deconstructive criticism
CONCRETE (focus on the behaviors that need to change) and with an element of *TEACHING* (it's clear what and how to change). For example, "You seem to have some difficulties in mathematics."	*GENERAL* (label globally and negative) and *ANTI-TEACHING* (it's not clear what or how to change). For example, "You are not worth teaching."
FOCUSED ON HOMEWORK: Doesn't judge but defines where the problem is. For example, "You seem to struggle the most with long division. In other parts of the math, you have no problem."	*FOCUSED ON THE PERSON:* Judges the person, rather than focusing on the task that wasn't done well. For example, "You're bad at math."
RESPECTFUL AND FRIENDLY TONE For example, "It happens to a lot of students."	*DISRESPECTFUL TONE* For example, "I don't know how you're such a mess. Your friends aren't like this."
BALANCED VIEW: Highlighting the aspects positives that are there as well. For example, "However in English, you're doing very well."	*FOCUSED ONLY ON THE NEGATIVE:* Not being able to recognize what the person is doing well. For example, "You do nothing right. You'll never be able to go to college."

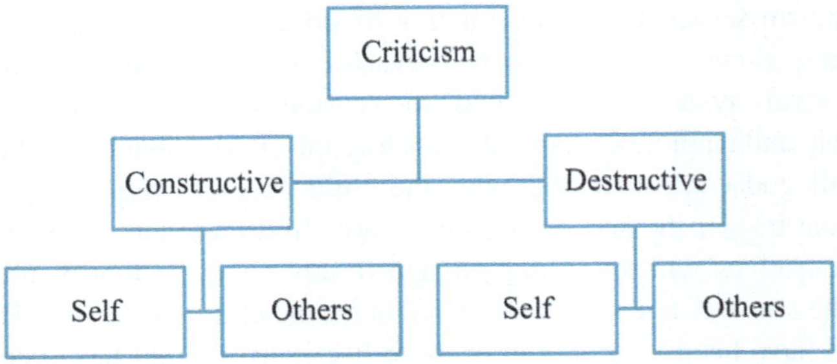

Fig. 5.1 Criticism diagram

How to Work with Destructive Self-Criticism: The Compassionate Voice

The way to work with the self-critical voice is to replace it with a compassionate inner voice. The practice of developing the figure of secure attachment, also called a compassionate friend, provides us with a loving, caring reference that will understand our mistakes and limitations. From someone like this, a compassionate and loving inner voice can emerge, which could have the same objectives as self-criticism but which will speak to us with another tone (compassionate instead of contemptuous or aggressive) and with other content (criticism will be constructive and not destructive). We'll help you develop the compassionate voice through different practices such as the "Letter to the Compassionate Friend," the practice of "Replacing the Critical Voice with Compassionate Voice," and "Developing the Secure Attachment Figure." These exercises will help you to gradually change the tone and the contents of your inner voice to a more compassionate, nonjudgmental one.

The Futility of Destructive Self-Criticism

Studies show that when we receive constructive criticism, we accept it better, we don't resist it as much, we set higher goals, and we feel more confident that we can achieve them. This is the reverse for destructive self-criticism. People with high destructive self-criticism don't achieve their goals as much as those with less destructive self-criticism. What's the reason?

Destructive self-criticism:

- It sets unrealistic goals.
- It makes us relentlessly evaluate ourselves, so we get discouraged. It decreases our motivation and increases our fear of failure.
- It prevents us from asking for help (because we feel inadequate), which also facilitates failure in interpersonal and romantic relationships.

For example, imagine a toddler who is learning to walk. If she falls down, she just gets back up. She's not engaging in destructive self-criticism by giving up or saying to herself "I'm not good at walking." The result? Eventually she learns to walk.

6 Formal Practice 2: Replacing the Critical Voice with Compassionate Voice

This practice is key in the shift toward having a more compassionate relationship with yourself. We recommend that you do the practice for a few weeks until it becomes habit.

And now, let's do the practice! (Supplementary Audio 5.2)

Also, you can find in the Annex 2 the practice in writing.

In addition to this formal practice, there are several ways to counteract the critical voice. You can decide on any of them or on a combination of several:

- Become aware and kindly counter the voice every time it appears. You can do this verbally without writing anything down. This is the most comfortable but the least effective way.
- Make a journal of the critical voice and see its evolution over time. This is the most time-consuming but also the most effective.
- Write weekly an example of the most destructive criticism of the critical voice, and see its evolution over time. This is an intermediate form in terms of effort and efficiency, so we highly recommend it.

7 Informal Practice 1: Letter from the Attachment Figure

The attachment figure tends to be a mix of "compassionate parent" and "wise teacher" who gives valuable advice and validates feelings.

The attachment figure shows great compassion and affection toward us with an idealized intensity not found in the real world. The attachment figure knows us perfectly, both the positive and negative aspects, and does not judge us because he or she knows the limitations of the human being. We know that our history has been key in the development of our current way of being, that we are all the product of our circumstances, and that our capacity for choice is limited. The attachment figure is not going to be "embarrassed" by the negative aspects it knows about us.

The compassionate letter is an expressive form of writing, which is known to be effective from a therapeutic point of view. The description of difficult events from a therapeutic perspective (in this case a compassionate perspective) helps us integrate and assimilate these experiences. The idea is to select a negative quality of your personality or a traumatic event that causes you shame or discomfort and write it as if it were written by someone (the attachment figure or compassionate friend) who perfectly understands what happens to us. The effect tends to be even greater if it is read a few days after being written. Sometimes it can be mailed and received a few days later, as if it came from someone else.

You can do this informal practice now, or you can do it as a homework assignment. To write the letter from the compassionate friend, follow the steps that are described as follows:

Letter from the Attachment Figure

Step 1: Pick something that makes you feel insecure, ashamed, or bad. It can be a characteristic, emotion, action, or whatever. Describe how you feel and what you tell yourself about it. You can be absolutely sincere since nobody is going to read it if you don't want them to.

Step 2: Imagine that the attachment figure/compassionate friend who knows you, understands, and cares unconditionally and that they write to you focusing on this topic, What do they care about?

What would they tell you about the "problem" from the perspective of their boundless compassion? How would they convey to you that what happens to you is simply human (shared humanity)? What suggestions do you think they would give you to better deal with those feelings? They write with the deepest compassion as someone who has infinite goodness. When you're done, save the letter (you can mail it), and read it several days later, as if it had not been written by you.

Here are some aspects that should be taken into account when practicing the letter to the attachment figure (Table 5.3).

The purpose of such letters is to identify and describe difficult feelings and situations and to develop acceptance for them to create more balanced and compassionate ways of working with the difficult feelings and situations. This is an ideal practice for working with feelings of shame.

Table 5.3 Aspects to take into account in the practice of the letter from the attachment figure

Is it free from judgments and not blaming?
Is it free from advice or "shoulds"?
Is there a tone of affection, compassion, and care?
Does it express real concerns for you?
Along with the content, the way it's said is very important. We recommend reading the letter to check if the tone is also compassionate.

Remember…

- Some of the specific mechanisms of action of compassion are as follows: reducing destructive self-criticism, reducing rumination, developing a new interpretation of negative life events, and regulating emotions.
- The efficacy of compassion is demonstrated in the treatment of anxiety and depression, as well as in other conditions involving stress and anger.
- Healthy people with self-compassion show more optimism, curiosity, creativity, and other positive emotions like enthusiasm and inspiration, compared to those more self-critical.
- The objective of compassion techniques is to improve the relationship that we have with ourselves, developing a secure attachment figure. The attachment figure is the core element of compassion.
- Self-criticism usually has two objectives: warning and feeling of control.
- The way to work with the self-critical voice is to replace it with a compassionate voice.

8 Self-Assessment Questions

You're doing very well! Now, let's review what you have learned in this module. For this, we will present you with a series of questions about the most important aspects. Don't worry if you don't know an answer; these questions are designed to help you.

Please Answer the Following Questions

	True	False
1. Some of the specific mechanisms of action of compassion are as follows: decreasing destructive self-criticism, decreasing ruminations, developing a new interpretation of negative life events, and regulating emotions.	T	F
2. The way compassion can be effective is by replacing negative thoughts and emotions with positive ones.	T	F
3. People with high destructive self-criticism don't achieve their goals as much as those with less destructive self-criticism.	T	F
4. One of the differences between constructive criticism and destructive criticism is that the former focuses on the task and the latter on the person.	T	F

Explanation of Self-Assessment Questions

Question	Correct answer	Explanation
1. Some of the specific mechanisms of action of compassion are the following: decreasing destructive self-criticism, decreasing ruminations, developing a new interpretation of negative life events, and regulating emotions.	T	As we have described above, there are two types of action mechanisms, those specific to compassion therapy and those that are common with mindfulness. Decreasing destructive self-criticism, decreasing ruminations, developing a new interpretation of negative life events, and regulating emotions are some of the specific mechanisms of action of compassion.
2. The way compassion can be effective is by replacing negative thoughts and emotions with positive ones.	F	The way compassion can be effective is not by replacing negative thoughts and emotions with positive ones but by embracing and accepting negative thoughts and emotions as part of human nature.
3. People with high destructive self-criticism don't achieve their goals as much as those with less destructive self-criticism.	T	People with high destructive self-criticism do not achieve their goals as much as those with less destructive self-criticism. Destructive self-criticism imposes unrealistic goals on us and causes us to relentlessly evaluate ourselves, so we get discouraged, decreasing motivation and increasing fear of failure. In addition, it prevents us from asking for help (because we feel inadequate), which also facilitates failure in interpersonal relationships.
4. One of the differences between constructive criticism and destructive criticism is that the former focuses on the task and the latter on the person.	T	Constructive criticism focuses on the task, does not judge the person, and defines what the problem is. For example, *You can tell a student: "You have the most difficulty with long division. In other parts of math, you have no problem."* Destructive criticism focuses on the person, judges them, and does not specify the task that is poorly done. (e.g., "You will never get anywhere.")

9 Homework

Next, we are going to present you with a series of tasks. As you already know, carrying out the tasks that we propose in each module is a fundamental pillar of this program. Remember, the more you know and practice, the more you can benefit from the online intervention. Therefore, in addition to reading, listening, and reviewing all the information that is included in each module, we ask you to put the homework into practice. Think of a toolbox that you go to when you have a problem. We are giving you valuable tools. Now you have to learn how to use them. And don't forget: The more time you put into learning the material and doing the exercises, the more you'll benefit from it.

In this module we ask you to perform the following tasks:

- Read the content of this module carefully, and review all the material it includes.
- Do Formal Practice 1 "Development of Attachment Figure" at least once. Depending on your situation, we recommend doing the practice several times a week on alternate days.
- Do Formal Practice 2 "Replace the Critical Voice with the Compassionate Voice" at least once. Depending on your situation, we recommend doing the practice several times a week on alternate days.
- In your daily life, try to identify and kindly refute your critical voice every time it appears.
- Write a weekly example of the most destructive criticism of critical voice, and observe its evolution over time.
- Write the "Letter from the Attachment Figure" if you have not already done so.
- Keep practicing the formal practice of "compassionate breathing" or "compassionate body scan" at least once a week each.
- Do any task/exercise/meditation we have recommended you and still have not done.

Congratulations! You have completed Module 3 "Developing Our Compassionate World."

In this module you have delved into the mechanisms of action of compassion, the attachment figure, and compassionate voice to increase your motivation and get involved in the practice, which can make it even more effective for you.

We encourage you to continue practicing everything you have seen in this module.

If you want, you can find the module summary in Annex 3. You can also download the audio of the formal practices of this module.

Annexes of the Module 3

Annex 1: Formal Practice 1 "Developmental Practice of the Attachment Figure"

Adopt the meditation posture that you usually use. Take a moment to observe the sensations that appear in your body, and take several deep breaths, with attention, to calm down and be able to let previous emotions and thoughts pass.

If you would like, you can start visualizing yourself in the safe place that you have developed in previous practices; visualize that place where you remember that you felt good, protected, and safe, and little by little, bring to mind the image of a real or imaginary person that constitutes your ideal model and the maximum expression of affection, wisdom, and compassion for you. You are looking for that person who represents these characteristics; if you don't know someone like this, you can make them up. You have to feel that this person transmits security and commitment to you and has the genuine desire for you to be happy and not experience suffering. On the other hand, you feel that you can tell them any aspect of your life, however negative it may be, because they will understand it without judging, even for things that you feel most ashamed about. This attachment figure that you are visualizing understands you, no matter what happens, and supports you unconditionally. The person has all the characteristics that you associate with well-being, understanding, affection, wisdom, and any other positive characteristic that is relevant to you. Stay for several seconds feeling these characteristics and thinking how they would be expressed in the attachment figure.

Think:

- What physical appearance (age, sex) would you want the attachment figure to have?
- How would they be dressed and in what environment would they be?
- What tone of voice would you want them to have?
- How would you like them to relate to you, and how would you want to relate to them?

Take a few minutes thinking about this, and you can also engage in this practice several times. When you have more or less defined the figure, it may progressively appear in front of you as if from a fog or an important place. Stay for a few moments being with your attachment figure. When you're ready, you can redirect your attention to your breath, letting go of any visual or mental phenomenon you experienced from this meditation, thus ending the practice.

Annex 2: Practice of Substituting the Critical Voice for the Compassionate Voice

The exercise is structured in three steps:

1. **First Step: Become Aware**

As cognitive therapy affirms, thoughts are more difficult to identify than feelings. On the other hand, the negative voice is part of our lives, and we are so used to it that we're not aware of it.

Therefore, it's easier to identify negative feelings and, later, identify negative thoughts.

To do this, in formal practice, identify a recent situation (last 6–12 months) where you felt bad. Reimagine the scene until you evoke the emotion you felt at that moment, and put a name to the emotion as you have already done in previous practices (fear, rage, anger, etc.). From there, listen for the self-critical voice. It is important to identify the exact words that the critical voice uses. That voice wants to help us, but with unhelpful methods. It's important to identify the exact criticism. If it is difficult for you to get up in the morning, the voice might say: "You are a lazy idiot" (insult and devalue you) or "You will never get there" (fear of failure) or "You disappoint me" (affective manipulation). It's important to see how that voice behaves, since the messages are going to repeat, and they will help you discover what your basic conflicts are in this area.

2. **Second step: responding with a compassionate voice**

We often respond to these critical voices by denying them and doing activities to avoid feeling them (e.g., eating, watching TV, listening to music, consuming substances, etc.). The other common response is to get angry (e.g., "Shut up!"), or we reprimand the person we think has given us that vision of the world (e.g., "It's like my dad is scolding me"). The answer must come from compassion. We must ask ourselves: "What would my attachment figure (or compassionate friend) say here?" It's like you are talking as the compassionate friend, trying to give yourself affection. The phrase can be something like, "I understand that you get angry [Use your own name here] because you think that this will accomplish something. But you have to understand that [your name] is exhausted, because she/he has been working hard for several months. It doesn't help her/him to criticize her/him because she/he will develop more feelings of inadequacy. Now [your name] must rest and recover." You can develop such a phrase based on what a compassionate friend would say about you.

3. **Third step: rely on the compassionate gesture to develop compassion**

Once you've developed the compassionate voice to counter the critical voice, you must evoke feelings of compassion to reinforce the speech. Therefore, you must emphasize with your body that compassionate feeling. The compassionate voice can be somewhat false if it is not coming from a compassionate place. That's why you must associate it with the self-compassionate gesture with which you have become familiar and stay with it for some time, feeling calm and comfortable with the experience.

Annex 3: Summary of the Module 3

Objectives of the Module

- Understand the mechanisms of action through which compassion works.
- Develop your own attachment figure, which is one of the core elements of compassion.
- Learn the types of disorders that compassion can be effective for.
- Learn what self-criticism is, the purpose it serves, as well as how to replace it with self-compassion.

Module Contents

How Compassion Works: Mechanisms of Action

(a) Specific mechanisms of compassion

✓ Decreasing self-criticism
✓ Decreasing rumination
✓Developing a new interpretation of negative life events
✓ Regulating emotions

(b) Mechanisms of action for the development of compassion specific to mindfulness

✓ Reduce affective biases through openness and psychological flexibility
✓ Increase open and curious nonreactive attention
✓ Regulation of emotions

The Attachment Figure

The attachment figure is the core element of compassion. It is the figure that can serve as a reference in situations of discomfort, difficulty, or doubt. The goal of compassion techniques is to improve the relationship that we have with ourselves, developing a secure attachment figure.

Compassion Efficacy

Self-compassion is considered effective in the treatment of anxiety and depression, as well as other psychiatric and medical conditions that involve stress and anger.

In healthy people, compassion is associated with psychological strengths such as:

- Emotional intelligence
- Wisdom
- Satisfaction with life
- Social connection
- Optimism
- Curiosity
- Creativity
- Enthusiasm
- Personal initiative
- Self-efficacy
- Intrinsic motivation
- Make changes that lead to self-improvement

The way to work with the self-critical voice is to replace it with a compassionate inner voice.

Self-criticism

Self-criticism is defined as criticism made by a person to oneself.

Types:

- Related to the feeling of inferiority and disappointment (this is the most common type).
- Related to self-hatred (occurs less frequently).

Goals:

- Warning: pay attention to something that makes us afraid
- Feeling of control

Homework

- Read the content of this module carefully, and review all the material it includes.
- Do Formal Practice 1 "Development of Attachment Figure" at least once. Depending on your situation, we recommend doing the practice several times a week on alternate days.
- Do Formal Practice 2 "Replace the Critical Voice with the Compassionate Voice" at least once. Depending on your situation, we recommend doing the practice several times a week on alternate days.
- In your daily life, try to identify and kindly refute your critical voice every time it appears.
- Write a weekly example of the most destructive criticism of critical voice, and observe its evolution over time.
- Write the "Letter from the Attachment Figure" if you have not already done so.
- Keep practicing the formal practice of "compassionate breathing" or "compassionate body scan" at least once a week each.
- Do any task/exercise/meditation we have recommended you and still have not done.
- Do any task/exercise/meditation we have recommended you and still have not done.

Chapter 6
Module 4: Understanding Our Relationship with Compassion

Module Objectives

In this module, we want to help you achieve the following goals:

- Learn and identify the biology behind compassion.
- Learn the attachment patterns and reflect on their importance in daily life.
- Become aware of your own attachment pattern that would explain how you function on an emotional level.
- Reflect on your ability to receive affection from friends, neutral people, and enemies.
- Receive affection from friends, neutral people, and enemies through formal practice.
- Understand the causes of guilt and learn to better handle this difficult emotion.
- Identify and describe the discomfort and difficult situations that have happened with your parents or caregivers, see the impact those experiences have on you now, and try to reconcile with your parents/caregivers to eliminate any remaining hatred or guilt toward them through the letter to parents.

Go ahead with the module. Don't feel like you need to hurry through it. It's more important to try to understand all the concepts that are presented and practice the exercises.

Module Contents

1. The Biology Behind Compassion
2. Attachment Patterns
3. Formal Practice 1: Become Aware of Our Attachment Pattern
4. The Importance of Attachment Patterns in Daily Life
5. Formal Practice 2: Capacity to Receive Affection: Friends, Neutral People, and Enemies

---

Supplementary Information The online version contains supplementary material available at https://doi.org/10.1007/978-3-031-38032-7_6.

J. García-Campayo et al., *The Attachment-Based Compassion Therapy*,
https://doi.org/10.1007/978-3-031-38032-7_6

6. Guilt
7. Formal Practice 3: Repairing Guilt
8. Relationship with Caregivers
9. Informal Practice: Letter to Parents or Caregivers
10. Self-Assessment Questions
11. Homework
12. Annexes

In this module, you will learn about the biology behind of compassion, the different patterns of attachment, and the importance of these patterns in daily life. You will start to identify your own pattern of attachment. These patterns develop early in life and can help explain our emotional functioning.

The meditation exercises in this module will help you receive affection from friends, enemies, and people who are neutral to you. Other practices in this module will help you identify and describe the difficulties you may have experienced with your parents/caregivers.

1 The Biology Behind of Compassion

Compassion is not only a psychological concept, or an abstract concept that only scientists and religious people use. Compassion is a measurable construct that can predict other things, like our overall well-being. Compassion is also based in biology.

There are several areas of the brain and a brain circuit associated with compassion. Compassion is closely tied to the way that we relate to other people, which is called our "attachment pattern."

Brain Circuits Related to Compassion

As a human, we have three key neurobiological systems (Gilbert, 2009). These systems or brain circuits are (1) satisfaction, calm, and security system, (2) threat and protection system, and (3) achievement system.

1. The satisfaction, calm, and security system: This system is the biological basis of our attachment patterns. It provides security, peace, and joy. It's activated in secure attachment relationships in the following ways:

   (a) For children, when they are hugged by their parents/caregivers and feel safe.
   (b) For adults, when they develop satisfactory, meaningful, and collaborative relationships.

   This system involves two neurotransmitters: endogenous opiates and oxytocin.

2. The threat and protection system: This system detects threats in the environment and makes us feel emotions like fear, anxiety, anger, and disgust. It can also be activated by thoughts we have, like fears about the future (of loss), self-criticism, or obsessive rumination. As humans, we lack the predators and survival threats we had in the past. However, this circuit is strongly activated by the social environment, which we can experience as threatening. This circuit is linked to the activity of adrenaline and cortisol.
3. The achievement system: This system pushes us to get food, to look for safe places to protect ourselves, and to find what is necessary for life. Modern society has more than met our survival needs (at least in developed countries). This means that now money, and everything it can buy, is used as a sign of status and is considered a main source of happiness. This continuous need for consumption over-activates the achievement system and is a major source of stress. This circuit is linked to the activity of dopamine.

Now that you know the different brain systems, think about how you experience them in today's society. Generally our threat system (e.g., self-criticism, shame) and our achievement system (e.g., consumerism, social status) are more activated, whereas our satisfaction, calm, and security system is less activated.

Compassion activates the satisfaction, calm, and security system, which is the only system able to offset the other two systems. This helps us return to tranquility and happiness.

2 Attachment Patterns

Compassion and Attachment Patterns: Attachment Theory

From an evolutionary point of view, compassion is key when caring for offspring in species like ours (and in mammals in general), because the young are very vulnerable at birth and require the intense care of adults for a long time to survive (Goetz et al., 2010). It is in these first years of life that we develop attachment, which is the capacity for affection and trust toward ourselves and other people.

Attachment theory, first developed by John Bowlby in 1969, argues that when children feel threatened, their attachment system is activated, and they instinctively seek caregiver protection.

When children find this kind of protection on a regular basis, they develop a "secure attachment." But if this protection fails, children can develop a deep insecurity in the relationship with their caregivers ("insecure attachment"). This insecurity can extend into their adult relationships as well, causing them to mistrust others. It can also have a negative impact on self-image. At that age, children cannot understand that their parents may not love them. Instead, children often think that they're doing something wrong and that when they know what it is and stop doing it, they will be loved again. Unfortunately, they often spend their entire childhood trying to understand why their parents do not love them, without succeeding.

Attachment theory is still considered one of the models that best describes the long-term dynamics of relationships between people. The theory proposes that children, in the first years of their life, need to develop a satisfactory, stable, and lasting relationship with at least one caregiver to have adequate psychological and emotional development. When children begin to crawl and walk away from their caregivers, they need the secure base provided by caregivers to explore the environment and return. This theory extends to attachment in adults as well.

Although some have criticized attachment theory as being too simplistic because it doesn't take into account other factors that affect attachment, such as temperament, it is still a widely accepted theory. In fact, it has been widely used in social protection policies for children to promote bonding with caregivers, and its principles are used in different types of therapy.

Attachment Styles

Early research categorized attachment into four types of patterns: a secure pattern and three insecure patterns (anxious, avoidant, and disorganized), each of which have different characteristics (Bartholomew & Horowitz, 1991).

These four categories of attachment were based on two factors – how we see ourselves (in a positive or negative way) and how we see other people (in a positive or negative way). The figure below shows that for each attachment category, we have either a positive or negative view of ourselves and a positive or negative view of others. Each type of attachment has a different way of relating to and communicating with others, as shown in the Fig. 6.1.

In Annex 1, you can find detailed information on the *types of attachment*, their characteristics, and main consequences.

More recently, researchers have begun to view attachment patterns as more of a continuum rather than a category. Research has found that people's attachment patterns vary along two dimensions: avoidance and anxiety (Fraley et al., 2015).

Attachment avoidance relates to how much we try to control our thoughts, feelings, and behaviors in relationships (e.g., allowing ourselves to open up to other people or depend on other people). People high in avoidance may fear being close to others and may feel that others are unresponsive to their needs. As a result, they may suppress their needs as a form of self-protection (Moreira et al., 2015). They may also struggle with intimacy in relationships, suppress their emotions, strive for emotional distance from others, and be overly self-reliant when they're distressed. They may withdraw from others to protect themselves from potentially being disappointed that the other person won't meet their needs (Mikulincer et al., 2003).

Attachment anxiety relates to how worried we are that someone will reject us. People high in anxiety may feel unworthy, clingy, and insecure about the

		Image you have of yourself	
		+	−
Image you have of others	+	**Secure (or trusting)** Positive view of self: Feeling worthy of the attention of others Positive view of others: Have confidence in and trust others	**Anxious** Negative view of self: Lacking confidence in self Positive view of others: Emotionally dependent on and trust others
	−	**Avoidant** Positive view of self: Compulsively self-confidence Negative view of others: Lack of confidence in and absolute mistrust in others	**Disorganized** Negative view of self: Lacking confidence in self Negative view of others: Fearful of intimacy and lack trust in others

Fig. 6.1 Type of attachmentNote: Prepared from Bartholomew and Horowitz (1991)

availability and responsiveness of others. They may be hypervigilant to signs of abandonment and rejection and seek ongoing reassurance from others, in part because they may be self-critical and doubt whether they deserve to have their needs met (Wei et al., 2011).

When people are low on attachment anxiety and avoidance, we describe them as being securely attached. People who are securely attached tend to hold a positive view of themselves and others and have higher self-worth, greater capacity for emotion regulation, and higher levels of interpersonal satisfaction and general well-being (Love & Murdock, 2004). People with this pattern expect that others will be available and respond to their needs in a supportive way (Mikulincer et al., 2003). This paves the way to positive psychological adjustment.

Although we can categorize people based on the avoidance and anxiety dimensions (as the Fig. 6.2 below shows), in reality our level of avoidance and anxiety in our relationships can be somewhere in the middle. In other words, someone can have moderate levels of avoidance and anxiety in relationships, rather than just high or low levels. These patterns of avoidance and anxiety vary along a spectrum and can also change over time.

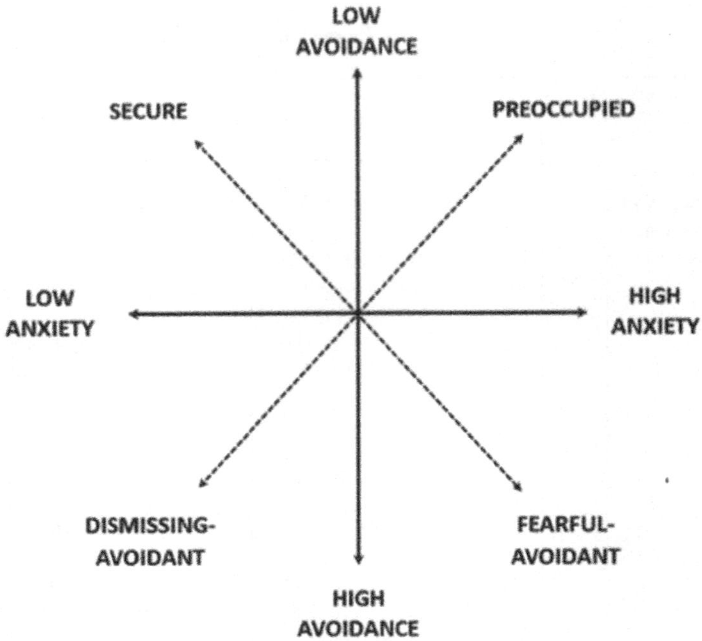

Fig. 6.2 Attachment patterns and avoidance and anxiety dimensions. (Source: Fraley et al., 2015)

3 Formal Practice 1: Become Aware of Our Attachment Pattern

Now that you know about attachment patterns and the way it can affect people's lives, it's time to look at your own attachment pattern. This exercise will help you identify the attachment pattern you developed as a child. We will also look at how it affects the way you approach relationships so that you can start to change the parts that may be causing suffering.

Listen to the audio below to do the formal practice of identifying your attachment pattern and becoming aware of how you relate socially as an adult (Supplementary Audio 6.1).

In Annex 2 you will find the instructions of the Formal Practice 1 to become aware and identify your own attachment pattern.

After the exercise, take some time to reflect on how you feel and the actions you take when you feel bad. You can think about this both for you now and for when you were a child.

Most people find that the behaviors are very similar in both cases, because the patterns we learn in childhood are the same ones we have as adults. Now that we have the connection with childhood, we can look at what our attachment pattern was like with our parents/caregivers.

4 The Importance of Attachment Patterns in Daily Life

Researchers estimate that 65% of children have a secure attachment pattern, and the other 35% have one of the insecure patterns described above (Prior & Glaser, 2006). The attachment pattern of the parents tends to predict the attachment pattern of the child 75% of the time (Steele et al., 1996).

Although there are other influences besides attachment, securely attached children are more likely to have better social skills than insecure ones. Secure attachment also helps with intellectual development and forming a social identity. Overall, there are a lot of benefits that come with having a secure attachment (e.g., Lee & Hankin, 2009; Tironi et al., 2021; Gumley et al., 2014; Cortés-García et al., 2019).

In general, people with a secure attachment function better at an interpersonal level and at other levels, like job performance. This is because our self-image and the impression we have of others influence almost all activities of daily life.

The most adverse attachment pattern is the disorganized one. Around 80% of newborns who suffered abuse fall into this group. Only about 15% of abused newborns are classified as securely attached. Children with a disorganized pattern in childhood tend to show disturbed relationship patterns in adulthood. These children are more likely to become abusive parents and suffer from psychiatric disorders in adulthood (e.g., Berlin et al., 2008).

In sum, attachment patterns influence the way we see ourselves and the way we see others. For example, it determines the level of shame or guilt we may feel or level of anger and mistrust we might have toward others. Attachment patterns are the key to the relationship we have with ourselves and with others.

Compassion is key to understanding and changing the relationship we have with ourselves and with others and is therefore closely related to attachment patterns.

5 Formal Practice 2: Capacity to Receive Affection: Friends, Neutral People, and Enemies

There are three main ways to experience compassion:

1. Receiving compassion or affection from others
2. Giving compassion to others
3. Giving yourself compassion

We need to be able to receive affection from others before we can give it. This stems from our survival as mammals. We are born vulnerable and unprotected, and we require the care of others to survive. If we understand our difficulties receiving affection, this will help us understand our difficulties giving it to others as well as to ourselves.

In the following formal practice, we will ask you to focus on receiving affection from friends, neutral people, and enemies. Try it out! (Supplementary Audio 6.2).

In Annex 3 you will find the transcript of the practice Capacity to Receive Affection: Friends, Neutral People, and Enemies.

After this practice, we recommend you reflect briefly on the difficulties you may experience in receiving affection from friends, neutral people, and enemies. The main topics for reflection are listed in Table 6.1.

Reflecting on these questions can help clarify your understanding of the points that are included below.

(a) Receive Affection from Friends

Healthy and compassionate people can easily ask for help when they need it because they are also willing to give it to others. If we can't accept help, others may not be as willing to accept help from us when we offer it. Healthy relationships have reciprocity.

Securely attached people do not feel they have to maintain any image of strength, since suffering, and the need for affection are common to all people (e.g., common humanity). Both receiving and giving affection are an expression of our connection with others. It can also create a feeling of happiness, even if the situation that requires help is difficult. The feeling of affection from others helps us overcome adversity.

(b) Receive Affection from Neutral People

Healthy and compassionate people have no problem receiving affection from people they don't know very well if they feel it's genuine. Securely

Table 6.1 Main topics of reflection in the practice of receiving affection from others

1. Receiving affection from friends
Are we capable of accepting affection from loved ones (even if we haven't asked for it)?
Are we capable of asking our loved ones for affection when we need it?
What does it mean for us to receive affection from others? (e.g., connection to others, weakness, debt of gratitude, etc.)
Do we have to maintain the image of being strong at any cost (and therefore we cannot allow ourselves to receive affection/help)?
2. Receiving affection from neutral people
Are we capable of receiving affection from people we don't know much about?
What does it mean for us to receive affection from these people?
What motivation do we feel these people have?
3. Receiving affection from enemies
Are we capable of receiving affection from people with whom we have a conflict?
What does it mean for us to receive affection from these people?
What motivation do we feel these people have?
Do we have to maintain an image that would be impacted if we accept help from them?

attached people don't think that these people have hidden agendas but (like themselves) tend to help people who need it. They see the situation as an opportunity to strengthen ties with people.

(c) Receive Affection from Enemies

Healthy and compassionate people have no problem receiving affection from people with whom they have a conflict if they feel it's genuine. They don't think that these people have hidden agendas but rather (like themselves) tend to help people who need it. They see the situation as an opportunity to strengthen ties and end the conflict. This desire is often the motivation for the other person to accept the help. They don't feel that they project an image of weakness for accepting help from someone with whom they have a conflict. Conflicts don't promote well-being and it's often better to resolve them, if possible.

6 Guilt

What Causes Guilt?

Guilt is the emotion that tells us that we have done something that goes against our moral code, such as the belief that we shouldn't hurt people. Therefore, we often feel guilt when we're convinced that we have caused someone harm. We tend to feel guilt when we have the thought, "I'm responsible for someone's misfortune," whether or not it's true.

Guilt can become harmful when we engage repetitively in the thinking patterns listed below:

- *Catastrophizing*: expecting the worst or most negative outcome in each situation.
- *Personalization*: blaming yourself for something you weren't entirely responsible for.
- *Overgeneralization*: viewing a negative event as a never-ending pattern of defeat.

Many people believe that if they don't feel guilty, then they are selfish or even a bad person. However, this is not the case.

Compassion makes us aware of the suffering of others and makes us want to reduce that suffering as much as we can. This emotion is much more prosocial than guilt and is associated with positive feelings.

The situations that usually produce guilt are:

Something you did, thought or felt.
Something you should have done, thought or felt.
Something you think you did.
Not helping someone enough.
Doing something better than other people.

How to Handle Guilt?

Some things that can help you better deal with guilt are the following:

- Have a flexible moral code (considering cultural and personal components) that makes sense to you.
- Don't have an idealized vision of yourself. That is, make yourself aware that you are human and that you will inevitably make mistakes. It's important to lower idealized standards about yourself that are impossible to meet.
- Avoid the "shoulds." These are rules that you continually demand of yourself and that, due to their very nature, are impossible to fulfill, since no human can always fulfill something. For example: "I should never be angry with my children."
- Understand that the origin of the feelings of guilt is based on your childhood. This is because you learned your moral code from your caregivers, educators, and environment. And it's your compliance or lack of compliance with this code that leads to feelings of guilt.
- Remember that guilt is not useful, it only increases suffering and decreases your effectiveness in helping others.

7 Formal Practice 3: Repairing Guilt

Here is a formal practice to work on guilt. If you are ready, you can listen to the following audio to do the practice of Repairing Guilt (Supplementary Audio 6.3).

In Annex 4 you will find the transcript of the practice *Repairing Guilt*.

8 Relationship with Parents/Caregivers

Parents (or our main caregivers if they were not present) are our main attachment figure. Our relationship with them creates the pattern that we use, unconsciously and repeatedly, in other relationships.

Understanding the type of relationship that you had with your parents will help you understand how you function in the present moment and what aspects you may try to change to reduce your suffering.

Relationships with parents are almost always conflictual. It is estimated that even the most competent parents are not available to their children 50% of the time due to work, housekeeping, personal issues, etc. (García-Campayo, 2019). Children's demand for affection is unlimited, but parental availability is not. Regardless of the time spent, the ability to give security and affection or to understand children's feelings is highly variable, not only between people but also throughout the life of the same person.

The *goal* of these compassion practices is not to look for culprits, but to identify the emotions you experienced during childhood. We want to understand the impact these childhood feelings have on your current relationship patterns to reduce your suffering.

9 Informal Practice: Letter to Parents/Caregivers

The letter is a form of expressive writing and is known to be therapeutic. Writing about conflicts in a compassionate way can help us integrate and assimilate these experiences. Here we ask you to use it as a homework assignment:

- In the letter you can express to your parents/caregivers (together or separately) the main emotions that they made you feel as a child, good and bad.
- It doesn't matter if your parents are alive or deceased, because this practice can help you resolve any resentment you may have toward them. To be clear, this letter is to help you reconcile for yourself any difficulties you had with your parents.
- It's not necessary (and sometimes it's counterproductive, like in cases of abuse) for this reconciliation to take place with your parents in real life.
- This internal reconciliation is independent from any potential legal issues with your parents (e.g., abusive situations). We recommend that you still do the exercise.

Below you can read the instructions for Informal Practice the Letter to Parents or Caregivers.

Step 1

Begin by writing about the good times with your caregivers, the positive aspects, the situations of care and affection that you've experiences with them, and any appreciation you feel for that affection. Try to write half of a page about this.

Step 2

Next, write about some of the bad moments with your caregivers: abandonment, misunderstanding, and punishment (in extreme cases, mistreatment). Describe how you feel and how you would have liked things to be. Also describe how you feel this has affected your current life. Try to write half of a page about this.

Step 3

Despite the bad times, write about your understanding of how your caregivers did the best they knew how to do at the time. There may have been other circumstances (e.g., hardships, their own personal history) that influenced their actions at the time. See if you can write about forgiving them and recovering the good times you had together. Understand that this is independent of whether you decide to see them anymore or not. Try to write half of a page about this.

Table 6.2 Things to consider when doing the Informal Practice Letter to Parents or Caregivers

Informal Practice Letter to Parents or Caregivers
Are positive aspects of the parents recognized and appreciated?
Can negative aspects be verbalized without hatred?
Can some of the problems of the present be linked to your relationship with your parents? (realistically)
Does the letter end with a tone of reconciliation and understanding?

See Table 6.2 for some things you can consider when you write the letter.

The goal of this letter is to (1) identify and describe the discomfort and difficult situations that you've experienced with your parents, (2) to see the impact those experiences have on you now, and (3) to be able to find reconciliation with your parents (even if you never verbalize these things to them in real life) so that you can remove any remaining hatred or blame toward them. We don't tend to feel hatred for someone when we don't expect a repair from that person or an explanation or request for forgiveness (even if we would like an apology).

Remember…

- Compassion is closely related to the way we relate to other people, also known as "attachment patterns." There are four main types of attachment in adults: secure attachment (trusting) and three insecure attachment patterns (anxious, avoidant, and disorganized).
- The main neurobiological systems or brain circuits are as follows: (a) satisfaction, calm, and security system, (b) threat and protection system, and (c) achievement system.
- The satisfaction, calm, and security system is activated in relationships with secure attachment. Identifying and being aware of your attachment pattern is key to knowing how it influences you in current relationships.
- There three main ways to experience compassion. These include (a) receiving compassion or affection from others, (b) giving compassion to others, and (c) giving compassion to oneself.
- Guilt arises because we are convinced that we have caused harm. This feeling is related to repetitive and dysfunctional thinking patterns characterized by catastrophizing, personalization, and overgeneralization.
- Understanding the type of relationship you had with your parents/caregivers will help you understand how you function at the current moment and what aspects you can try to modify to reduce your suffering.
- The objective of compassionate practices is not to look for culprits but to identify the emotions that we had in childhood, how they impact our current relationships, and the ways we can modify the patterns to reduce our suffering.

10 Self-Assessment Questions

You're doing very well! Now, let's review what you have learned in this module. For this, we will present you with a series of questions about the most important aspects. Don't worry if you don't know an answer; these questions are designed to help you learn.

Please answer the following questions:

	True	*False*
1. Of the three brain circuits, the achievement system is the one related to compassion.	T	F
2. Attachment patterns influence the image we have of ourselves and of others; therefore, they are the key to the relationship we have with ourselves and with others.	T	F
3. Secure attachment is characterized by a caregiver responding in an inconsistent way – at times having an appropriate response and other times, an inappropriate response.	T	F
4. The "avoidant" attachment pattern is characterized by having a positive self-image (excessively self-confident) and a negative self-image of others (excessively distrustful of others).	T	F

Explanation of Self-Assessment Questions

Question	Correct answer	Explanation
1. Of the three brain circuits, the achievement system is the one related to compassion.	False	The achievement system encourages us to get food, to look for safe places to protect ourselves, and to find what is necessary for life. Compassion allows the activation of the satisfaction, calm, and secure system, which helps us restore tranquility and happiness and counteracts the over-activation produced by the other two systems.
2. Attachment patterns influence the image we have of ourselves and of others; therefore, they are the key to the relationship we have with ourselves and with others.	True	That's right! The attachment patterns that have developed in your childhood serve as the basis for the social relationships that you establish as an adult.
3. Secure attachment is characterized by a caregiver responding in an inconsistent way – at times having an appropriate response and other times, an inappropriate response.	False	This is false and corresponds to disorganized attachment pattern. Secure attachment is characterized by experiences of adequate childcare, safety, and affection provided consistently and continuously.

Question	Correct answer	Explanation
4. The avoidant attachment pattern is characterized by having a positive self-image (excessively self-confident) and a negative self-image (excessively distrustful of others).	True	Right! As a consequence of childhood experiences of inadequate or inconsistent care, excessive self-confidence and extreme distrust of others develops, based, in part, on this exaggeratedly positive image of themselves and the negative vision of others.

11 Homework

Next, we are going to present you with a series of tasks. As you already know, carrying out the tasks that we propose in each module is a fundamental pillar of this program. Remember, the more you know and practice, the more you can benefit from the online intervention. Therefore, in addition to reading, listening and reviewing all the information that is included in each module, we ask you to put the homework into practice. Think of a toolbox that you go to when you have a problem. We are giving you valuable tools. Now you have to learn how to use them. And don't forget: The more time you put into learning the material and doing the exercises, the more you'll benefit from it.

In this module we ask you to perform the following tasks:

- Read the content of this module carefully, and review all the material it includes.
- Do Formal Practice 1 "Become Aware of Our Attachment Pattern" at least once. If possible, we recommend doing the practice several times a week on alternate days.
- Do Formal Practice 2 "Capacity to Receive Affection: Friends, Neutral People, and Enemies" at least once. If possible, we recommend doing the practice several times a week on alternate days.
- Do Formal Practice 3 "Repairing Guilt" at least once. If possible, we recommend doing the practice several times a week on alternate days.
- Do the Informal Practice "Letter to Parents or Caregivers."
- Observe and become aware of how the attachment pattern plays out in your daily life.
- Use the Compassion Practice Journal to record your meditative practice.
- Keep practicing the Formal Practice of "Compassionate Breathing and Compassionate Body Scan" at least once a week each.
- Review any previous modules that you have questions about.
- Do any task/exercise/meditation that we have recommended and you have not already done.

Congratulations!! You have completed Module 4 "Understanding Our Relationship with Compassion."

In this module you have delved into the biology behind compassion, attachment patterns, and the importance of these patterns in daily life.

We encourage you to continue practicing everything you have seen in this module. Keep going; you're more than halfway through the intervention!

If you'd like, you can find the module summary in Annex 5.

You can also download the audio of the formal practices of this module.

Annexes of the Module 4

Annex 1. Attachment Styles

- *Secure (or Trusting) Attachment Pattern*: These are individuals who experienced adequate childcare that is consistent and continuous. That is why they developed confidence in themselves and in others. As a result, people with a secure attachment style tend to like themselves and feel worthy of affection. They also feel comfortable depending on other people, so they can request help from others and be confident that they'll receive it when they need it. There is a balance between emotional needs and personal autonomy.
- *Anxious Attachment Pattern*: These are individuals who experienced variable care as a child, where the response from their caregiver fluctuated between adequate care and absent care. This means that care has been erratic and unstable, where the child would randomly receive care, or not, usually depending on the levels of pathology or adverse circumstances of the caregiver at any given moment. For example, this pattern has been found in children of parents with bipolar disorder, frequent depression, or illnesses that appear intensely in cyclical periods (e.g., migraine or rheumatological diseases). The consequence is that people with this pattern put a lot of weight on the opinion of others on whom they depend. Because they tend to have a negative view of themselves, they give up any of their wishes or goals if they conflict with the approval of others. They tend to have low self-esteem, high dependence on others, high subjective stress, and a focus on negative thoughts and feelings. They have continuous worry about being abandoned, which can cause problems in their relationships.
- *Avoidant Attachment Pattern*: These are individuals who have experienced a consistently inadequate or absent response from their caregiver when they were a child. In contrast to the anxious attachment pattern, people with this pattern have never experienced adequate care. This pattern often occurs when caregivers have addictions, personality disorders, or psychosomatic diseases, such as hypochondriasis or severe somatizations, which force them to focus all of their attention on themselves, leaving no room for caring for others. For this reason, this group of people develops absolute distrust of others and compensate by depending entirely on themselves. Although their vision of others is negative due to their experiences as children, they tend to have an exaggeratedly positive view of themselves

and excessive self-confidence. In their relationships with others, they tend to look down on the need for affection from others. They view this as a weakness because they learned to survive independently without anyone's help. In fact, they tend to be the most likely to reject compassion. They tend to be achievement oriented, with few emotional needs and few significant interpersonal relationships. However, they are very emotionally self-sufficient, so the lack of interpersonal intimacy doesn't necessarily bother them.

- *Disorganized Attachment Pattern*: These are individuals who have suffered from a frightening or violent response from their caregiver, based on rejection or punishment. This pattern is common when parents are abusive, alcoholic, or substance-dependent or have serious mental or personality disorders. They tend to have a very negative view of both others and of themselves. Children, in these cases, don't understand that their parents have a disorder but instead think that they are doing something wrong and that is why they are punished. The consequence is that throughout childhood they try to understand what they did wrong and try to change so that their caregiver doesn't hit or mistreat them but without success. Like those with the anxious attachment pattern, they have low self-esteem and a negative view of themselves. Although they desire social contacts, they suppress this desire because of fear of rejection. Their interpersonal relationships as adults are characterized by running away after reaching a certain degree of intimacy. They usually consider personal relationships as secondary to their work or professional goals.

Annex 2. Practice of Identifying Your Own Attachment Pattern

Adopt the meditation posture that you usually use, and stay there for a few moments observing the bodily sensations that appear, the contact of the feet with the ground, and take several deep breaths, with attention, so that you can let previous emotions and thoughts just pass.

Little by little bring to your mind some recent situation that happened in the last 6–12 months where you felt bad. Choose a situation that was a moderate level of emotional intensity.

Once you have a situation in mind, remember it as accurately as possible (what you were doing, who you were with, what you said, and what the other person told us, etc.), and evoke the emotion you felt in that moment, so that you can label it later on. Now that you've put yourself back in that situation, remember how you tended to react in that moment: what did you say to yourself (what was your internal dialogue)? What did you do (isolate yourself, talk to someone, and if so, what did you talk about and with whom, etc.)? Remember the whole process of how you coped with that situation of discomfort.

Little by little, try to summarize in a short phrase what you think and what you do when you feel bad (e.g., when something bad happens to me, I think that I am useless and will never be able to overcome my defects. I tend to withdraw from others because I fear being questioned or feeling rejected). If you have been able to summarize that phrase, return to your breath for a few seconds, and let any thoughts and emotions that have appeared to pass.

Now think of a situation that happened when you were a child (sometime between the ages of 6–14) and you felt bad. As before, it should be a situation of moderate intensity, not the greatest trauma of your life, but something that you can focus on. Once you've chosen the situation, try to rebuild it from memory in the most accurate way possible (e.g., how your life was, what you were doing at the time, who you were with, what you said and what the other person told you, how that feeling of discomfort came about, etc.). Remember everything you can until you can feel the emotion you felt at the time. Now that you feel it, connect with that feeling of discomfort, and label it, identifying what kind of emotion it was (sadness, fear, anger, etc.). How did you react at that moment: What did you say to yourself? What did you do? Remember what role your parents or caregivers played when you felt bad. Did you look to them for protection? Did you tell them how you felt or not? What was your relationship with them in those moments of discomfort?

Summarizing all that you remember, construct a small phrase about what you thought and did when you were a child when you felt bad and what support you had from your caregivers at that time. A phrase like,

"When I was little and I felt bad, I thought I was weird; I tried to tell my parents, but they always told me they didn't have time for my nonsense."

Once you have the phrase, return to your breath for a few seconds, and let the thoughts and emotions that have been appeared during this exercise just pass.

Finally, in the third part of this exercise, think about what your general relationship was like with your caregivers or parents. If you had two parents or caregivers, your relationship with each person may be different. Did you feel safe when you were afraid? Protected by them? Did you feel loved and supported in any circumstance? Could you express your feelings because you knew you were going to be listened to and valued?

Try to summarize and identify your relationship with each caregiver in three aspects: (1) security and fear, (2) feeling loved and supported, and (3) how much you felt they understood you when you expressed your feelings. It's possible you experienced some changes in your parents during your childhood, especially if some important event occurred during that time: some loss, some separation, or other important event. With all this in mind, make a small phrase summarizing how you felt in the relationship with your caregivers. If it was different for each caregiver, you can create two separate phrases. (e.g., "Although my mom was good to me, I used to perceive her as distant, with little time to listen to me or to worry about the things that happened to me or how I felt"). Stay a few moments with this phrase or separate phrases if it was different for each caregiver.

Now that you've done all three exercises, try to make a connection between them, with how you act in the present, how you acted when you were little, and what your relationship was like with your caregivers. See if there is any connection, some commonality, or some aspect that catches your attention. Spend a few moments trying to understand all this. When you feel ready, little by little, focus your attention to your breathing for a few seconds, letting go of any thoughts or emotions that you may have had during this practice. When ready, you can return to your body, move your arms and legs, open your eyes, and end the exercise.

Annex 3. Practice Receiving Affection from Friends, Neutral People, and Enemies

Adopt the meditation posture that you usually use. Dedicate a few moments to feel your body and take several deep breaths, with attention, so that you can let previous emotions and thoughts just pass.

Little by little, begin to bring to mind some recent situation (within the last 6–12 months) of mild or moderate intensity in which you felt bad. Remember the circumstance as clearly as possible (what you did, who you were with, what you said and what the other person said, etc.), until you evoke the emotion you felt in that moment. Connect with the emotion and put a label on it.

Now that you're feeling the discomfort of that situation, imagine a situation in which you felt similarly (e.g., bad) and someone you love and you have affection for (e.g., partner, family, friends, etc.) offered you help; it can be help of any kind: emotional, financial, etc. Remember a situation in which this happened (or if it has never happened to you, imagine what it would be like to receive help from a loved one). Imagine how the situation might unfold and observe how you respond in that situation: What do you feel and what do you say to yourself when you receive help from a loved one? What does that mean to you? Do you see it as positive reinforcement in that it makes you feel good and flattered, or does it make you feel bad because you're concerned it makes you look weak or vulnerable?

Connect with what you feel, with what you think and with what you do in these moments. Do you accept or not accept the help? Do you grudgingly accept it? Do you run away from that person so they don't have to help you? There are many options. Observe how you tend to behave in these types of situations. Think of a small phrase to summarize it: When I feel bad and someone who loves me offers me his help, I think and feel (fill in the blank) and I end up reacting as follows….

Once you've created the phrase, turn your attention back to the breathing, letting thoughts and feelings pass for a few seconds. Little by little return again to the situation in which you felt bad. Imagine (or if it has actually happened to you, recall the specific situation) that someone you don't know very well (a co-worker from another division, a neighbor, a friend of a friend, etc.) learns that you're having a hard time and offers you help or support. Observe: What do you feel, and what do you tell yourselves when you get help from someone you don't know? Can you accept this help or not? What image do you have of yourself and of the other person if you accept? Would you distrust it and think it's ridiculous that the person would actually want to help? How would you react? Think of a small phrase to summarize it: If someone I don't know very well offers me help, I would think and feel (fill in the blank) and I would react as follows….

Refocus your attention on your breath, and spend a few seconds letting go of your thoughts and feelings.

Return to the situation in which you felt bad. Imagine that someone you don't get along with (former partner, family member or former friend, etc.) learns that you're having a hard time and offers you help or support. Observe: What do you feel and what do you tell yourself when you get help from someone you don't get along with? Do you think about what could help you get closer to this person? Do you distrust the help of this person? Does it make you feel inferior, or, on the contrary, does it make you feel good? Would you accept the help or not?

Stay here for a few moments, identifying what you would think, what you would feel, and you would do. Think of a small phrase to summarize it: If I felt bad and someone I don't get along with offered me their help, I would think and feel (fill in the blank) and I would end up reacting in the following way….

To finish, turn your attention again to your breath and stay here a few moments so that you can let the thoughts and emotions from this practice just pass. Little by little, return to your body, move your arms and legs, open your eyes, and end the exercise.

Annex 4. Formal Practice Repairing Guilt

Get into a comfortable position, sitting or lying down, letting your body rest and stabilize. Take a couple of deep breaths becoming aware of any bodily sensations that arise. And keep breathing in and out.

Little by little begin to bring to mind the different events or situations when you have felt guilty. And try to get to the origin of this guilt. When did you feel it for the first time? This feeling is closely related to how critical our parents were of us when we were little and our own expectations for ourselves. Notice how this emotion developed for you and the role it played in different situations.

Now, choose a key moment in your life where guilt was present. And think back to what started it: it could be infidelity, not being with your parents at the time of their death, or anything you did that you think was a mistake. If you notice that tension appears in your body, invite the area in which you feel it to relax. And keep breathing in and out.

Connect with the negative evaluation you make of yourself when guilt appears. What thoughts lead you to feel this way? Become aware of them. The blame arises because you punish yourself harshly by judging your actions inflexibly. Does this really help you?

Just try to accept this feeling, being aware of why it appears, but without criticizing yourself for it. Accept that mistakes are part of being human and that guilt only lives in you. It's just an imaginary idea that you have built yourself based on your own expectations and those that others have of you. But it is not a reality.

And placing your hands on your heart, breathe in and out deeply, as a symbol of affection and acceptance toward yourself. Feel when you breathe in like your whole body is filled with energy, a special and restorative energy that takes care of you and reassures you. Let that energy flood everything, reduce the intensity of your thoughts, criticisms, and "shoulds," and connect with all the goodness and love that is in you.

Understand that any action carried out was the best you could do in each moment based on your history and the experience that you had at that point in life. In each breath out, allow your guilt to fade and progressively thin.

Stay in this state for as long as you need. When you're ready, become aware of your surroundings, and begin to move your body ending the practice.

Annex 4. Summary of the Module 4

Module Objectives

- Learn and identify the biology behind compassion.
- Learn the attachment patterns and reflect on their importance in daily life.
- Become aware of your own attachment pattern, which helps explain how you function on an emotional level.
- Reflect on your ability to receive affection from friends, neutral people, and enemies.
- Receive affection from friends, neutral people, and enemies through formal practice.
- Understand the causes of guilt and learn to better handle this difficult emotion.
- Identify and describe the discomfort and difficult situations that have happened with your caregivers; see the impact those experiences have on you now. Try to reconcile with your caregivers to eliminate any remaining hatred or guilt toward them through the Informal Practice Letter to Parents or Caregivers.

Module Contents

Biology Behind Compassion The three neurobiological systems or brain circuits related to compassion are the following:

- The satisfaction, calm, and security system
- The threat and protection system
- The achievement system

Compassion allows the activation of the satisfaction, calm, and security system which is the only one capable of counteracting over-activation of the other two systems, which then allows you to restore tranquility and happiness.

Attachment Patterns Compassion is closely related to the basic way we relate to other people, which is called our "attachment pattern." There are four types of attachment patterns in adults: secure, anxious, avoidant, and disorganized.

The Importance of Attachment Patterns in Daily Life Attachment patterns influence how we view ourselves and others; so identifying and being aware your attachment pattern is key to knowing how it influences you in current relationships with other people.

Guilt We feel guilt when we're convinced that we've have caused someone harm. It's related to repetitive and dysfunctional thinking patterns characterized by catastrophizing, personalization, and overgeneralization.

Relationship with Parents/Caregivers Caregivers are our main attachment figure, and our relationship with them creates the pattern we use in the rest of our relationships. Understanding the type of relationship you had with your parents/caregivers will help you understand how you function at the current moment and what aspects you can try to modify to reduce your suffering.

Homework Read the content of this module carefully, and review all the material it includes.

- Do Formal Practice 1 "Become Aware of Our Attachment Pattern" at least once. If possible, we recommend doing the practice several times a week on alternate days.
- Do Formal Practice 2 "Capacity to Receive Affection: Friends, Neutral People, and Enemies" at least once. If possible, we recommend doing the practice several times a week on alternate days.
- Do Formal Practice 3 "Repairing Guilt" at least once. If possible, we recommend doing the practice several times a week on alternate days.
- Do the Informal Practice "Letter to Parents or Caregivers."
- Observe and become aware of how the attachment pattern plays out in your daily life.
- Use the Compassion Practice Journal to record your meditative practice.
- Keep practicing the Formal Practice of "Compassionate Breathing and Compassionate Body Scan" at least once a week each.
- Review any previous modules that you have questions about.

Do any task/exercise/meditation that we have recommended and you have not already done.

Chapter 7
Module 5: Working on Ourselves

Module Objectives
In this module, we want to help you achieve the following goals:

- Understand the importance of affection (or compassion) towards yourself and towards others, and learn how this will help you create a secure attachment pattern.
- Do the Formal Practice "Giving Affection to Friends and Neutral People."
- Do the Formal Practice "Giving Ourselves Affection."
- Learn the causes of shame and to learn how to handle this difficult emotion.
- Do the Formal Practice "Reconciliation with Parental Figures," and reflect on the difficulties and different emotions with the practice.
- Identify Three Positive and Three Negative Things About Your Parental Figure(s) through a practical exercise, to continue reflecting on the relationship you've had with them.
- Do Informal Practice 1 "The Greatest Show of Affection Ever Received"
- Reflect on how we usually classify people into three categories: friends, enemies, and neutral people. Giving affection can be easier or more difficult depending on the category in which we've place the person.

Go ahead with the module. Don't feel like you need to hurry through it. It's more important to try to understand all the concepts that are presented and practice the exercises.

Module Contents
1. Importance of Affection Towards Ourselves and Towards Others
2. Formal Practice 1: Give Affection to Friends and Neutral People
3. Formal Practice 2: Giving Ourselves Affection
4. Shame

Supplementary Information The online version contains supplementary material available at https://doi.org/10.1007/978-3-031-38032-7_7.

J. García-Campayo et al., *The Attachment-Based Compassion Therapy*,
https://doi.org/10.1007/978-3-031-38032-7_7

5. Formal Practice 3: Repairing Shame
6. Formal Practice 4: Reconciliation with Parental Figures
7. Exercise 1: Three Positives and Three Negatives About Your Parental Figures
8. Informal Practice 1: The Greatest Show of Affection Ever Received
9. Self-Assessment Questions
10. Homework
11. Annexes

In this module we will focus on the importance of affection towards yourself and towards others. This will help you rebuild (or consolidate) your attachment pattern towards a secure attachment. We will also explore the emotion of shame. Below, you will find theoretical information, exercises, and formal and informal practices to help you continue working on yourself.

1 Importance of Affection Towards Ourselves and Towards Others

Before moving forward, it is important to identify and recognize what your attachment pattern is. It is possible that you have characteristics of several of them, although there is usually one that stands out.

- If your main pattern is secure attachment, it will be easier for you to practice compassion. This is because affection and compassion are natural parts of secure attachment. Therefore, you can aim to practice, remember, and assimilate what you've learned about the compassion-based intervention.
- If your attachment pattern is different from secure attachment, it may require more work and training. This is because you likely haven't had as much experience with affective or compassion.
- Specifically, if your pattern is fearful attachment, and there has been some form of abuse, you may benefit from additional therapy. In addition to engaging in the compassion-based intervention, we recommend consulting with a mental health professional.

The main difference between the secure pattern and the insecure patterns is the relationship you have with yourself and with others. It is crucial to be aware of this if you are looking to change the insecure attachment pattern to a secure one or reinforce/consolidate the secure pattern.

Relationship broadly refers to what we think, what we feel, how we act, and what expectations we have of ourselves and of others. The attachment pattern isn't just about an "image" we have of ourselves and others. Instead, it involves our thoughts, feelings, actions, and expectations.

In this intervention, we are going to use words to help you develop compassion. Words are very powerful. You probably can remember insults or painful criticisms that you've received. The impact of these words can stay with us for a long time.

The words you say to yourself (i.e., your internal dialogue) change how you think and feel. That's why it's very important to use compassionate language with yourself. Here we'll use kind and compassionate words, visualized images, attention-concentration, connection with others, and self-care to help you become more affectionate towards yourself and others.

Usually, it's easier to start by giving affection to others and then work on giving affection to ourselves. It can be harder to give affection to ourselves because it can make us feel guilty or selfish.

2 Formal Practice 1: Give Affection to Friends and Neutral People

In the same way that we categorize things into groups of what we like, what we don't like, and what we're indifferent about, we do the same with people. We call them friends, enemies, and neutral people.

It's easiest to express affection/compassion to friends (e.g., partner, family, friends, coworkers, and all the people with whom we have an emotional bond).

It can be more difficult to express affection to people classified as neutral people. That is, people you don't know intimately and with whom you have no special emotional ties (e.g., an acquaintance, a friend of a friend, the person who brings you the mail, etc.).

It's the most difficult to express affection to enemies, which includes not just declared enemies (which you may not have), but also people with whom you have conflicts of any kind, who have disappointed you, or with whom the relationship has deteriorated for whatever reason. We will work on this third category separately, in what we call advanced compassion, since it's somewhat more difficult. Broadly speaking, it would mean recognizing that, like you, they have fears, worries, hardships, and experience suffering. This is what makes us all equal as humans.

In the following Formal Practice (Annex 1), we encourage you to work on affection towards friends and neutral people. Go ahead!

After practicing, we recommend briefly reflecting on the difficulties that have emerged in expressing affection to friends and neutral people (Supplementary Audio 7.1).

To help you with this exercise, we suggest some things to consider in the Table 7.1 below.

In both cases, you may find you give affection in a similar way as your parents did (or main caregivers). The goal is not to find culprits but to find solutions and understand these patterns. Once you identify this, you can modify your emotional responses to reduce your suffering and increase your well-being.

> People with secure attachment can spontaneously give affection (they don't need to be asked to do so). They don't feel bad for giving affection, and they don't feel vulnerable. These people are also capable of giving affection to unknown people simply because they are suffering.

Table 7.1 Main topics of reflection in the practice of giving affection to friends and neutral people

1. Giving affection to a friend	Can you spontaneously give your loved ones affection, or do they have to ask you for it? When you give affection to your loved ones, do you feel bad, or do you resist for any reason? Do you express affection physically and, if so, how? What do you think of yourself when you give affection? (e.g., do you feel vulnerable or dependent?)
2. Giving affection to a neutral person	Can you give affection to a person you don't know at all, simply because they are suffering? How do you feel when you give affection to someone you don't know? (e.g., stupid, suspicious, confident, calm, proud, etc.) Do you express affection physically and, if so, how?

3 Formal Practice 2: Giving Ourselves Affection

Once you have been able to give affection to loved ones and neutral people, you can move on to giving affection to yourself. For most people it's more difficult to give affection to yourself than to others.

For some people this practice is very difficult. It may be hard because they experience it as a weakness or a risk of becoming vulnerable. For others, they find it hard because they don't consider themselves worthy of receiving affection.

In this case, a good strategy is to start the practice by giving affection to friends. When you are giving affection to people you love, you can include yourself in the image and give affection to yourself as well. This is easier because you aren't giving affection only to yourself (which is usually more difficult) but to yourself and the people you love at the same time (Supplementary Audio 7.2).

In Annex 2 you will find the transcription if the practice "Giving Ourselves Affection".

After practicing, we recommend that you reflect for a moment on the difficulties you may have in giving yourself affection. We suggest some topics for reflection.

- Can you give yourself affection spontaneously, or does it seem unnatural to you? If emotions are generated, how are these emotions felt in your body?
- What do you think when you give yourself affection, what resistance do you have? (Do you feel that you become a lazy, unsuccessful, careless person?)
- Would you give affection to a small child who was crying but insult and criticize yourself if you were feeling bad? If so, what is the logic behind this way of behaving?

People with secure attachment can spontaneously give themselves affection as often as they need it. They don't feel bad or guilty about it. They can treat themselves when they suffer as they would treat a small child who was crying. Sometimes, when we feel bad, we regress emotionally, and our most childish side comes out, seeking protection and understanding.

> Remember: You can be a good attachment figure for yourself (although not necessarily the only one).

4 Shame

Our main desire as humans is to be loved. This is why we often feel the need to belong to a group: family, friends, or other groups (work, hobbies, religious, neighborhood, etc.). Shame controls our behavior. The fear of being expelled from the group, or rejected, motivates us to follow the rules.

> Shame is an *unpleasant* emotion that is associated with feelings of inferiority, destructive self-criticism, hiding behaviors to avoid conflict with the group, and isolation.

In general, there are two types of shame:

(a) External: What you think others think of you and imagining that they think negatively of you.
(b) Internal: Something about you that is "unspeakable." Something that if the others knew, you think they would reject you. Informally, these fears are called "skeletons in the closet." This is the biggest barrier to connecting with others.

Compassion helps us reduce shame. Some practices to work on shame are the "Letter to the Compassionate Friend," "Forgiving Yourself," and "Repairing Shame."

Shame and guilt are related, but they are different. Guilt focuses on specific behaviors and compels you to apologize or repair the damage you caused. Shame is global, focusing on the whole person and making you feel inferior. In both cases, you may react by denying the action, shifting the blame onto another person, or being aggressive.

5 Formal Practice 3: Repairing Shame

Here is the Formal Practice of *Repairing Shame* that will help you work with this emotion (Supplementary Audio 7.3).

In Annex 3 you will find the instructions of the formal practice of Repairing Shame.

6 Formal Practice 3: Reconciliation with Parental Figures

Parents (or caregivers) are the key figures in the development of our attachment patterns. Therefore, they've greatly influenced our current social relationships and relationship we have with ourselves.

Almost everyone has had some conflict at some point with their parents or main caregiver.

Parents can't always meet our expectations. They can't always be fair and affectionate. Even the best parents make the wrong decisions sometimes. They don't spend as much time as they would like with their children or are angry or critical at times. So, reconciling with your parental figure, whether in real life or not, is one of the most healing practices in compassion-based interventions.

If your parental figure was abusive, toxic, or greatly harmful to you, you may want to skip the Formal Practice 3 "Reconciliation with Parental Figures" until you feel ready. It is also ok if you never feel ready. The reconciliation is meant to be done on your own, for yourself. We don't recommend that you reach out to the abusive person to try to reconcile with them in real life. However, this exercise may help you have a better understanding of this person and reduce any hatred or resentment you may feel. Holding onto hatred or resentment is harmful to your physical and psychological health, so letting go of these feelings will ultimately benefit you.

You can try it now, or, if you prefer, you can choose to do the practice at another time (Supplementary Audio 7.4).

In Annex 4 you will find the transcription of the formal practice "Reconciliation with Parental Figures."

Once you do the practice, we recommend that you reflect on the difficulties and feelings that you experienced.

7 Exercise 1: Three Positives and Three Negatives About Your Parental Figures

Next, try writing down three good things that you received from your parental figures (e.g., father/mother) throughout your life. You can write them for both of your parental figures or for each one separately. Also write down three negative aspects that you wish you could have changed or improved about your relationship with them.

You can use the following template:

Three Positives and Three Negatives About Your Parental Figure(s)
The following exercise consists of writing down three good things that you have received from your parental figure(s) throughout life. If you have two parental figures, you can write these things about both of them together or each one separately. Next write down three negative aspects that you wish you could have changed or improved about your relationship with them.

Three positive things about your parental figure(s)

1. ....
2. ....
3. ....

Three negative things about your parental figure(s)

1. ....
2. ....
3. ....

After you're done, it's important that you reflect on the exercise:

- There are people who can only see the negative aspects of their parents. If this is your case, we recommend you try to identify the positive aspects to balance your perspective of them and begin the reconciliation process.
- On the other hand, there are people who are unable to see a single negative thing about their parents. This happens when we idealize our parents and don't allow ourselves to think anything negative about them because we feel bad or guilty. In this case, it's important to recognize that it's common to find negative aspects since your parents are human. Because of this, they aren't perfect and will have their weaknesses. If you can't find negative aspects of your parents, it could negatively impact your romantic and social relationships because no partner or friend can be as perfect as your idealized parents.

8 Informal Practice 1: The Greatest Show of Affection Ever Received

When you have free moments throughout the day, we encourage you to think about the greatest display of affection you have ever received from another person. There may be several and it may be difficult to identify which is the greatest. It's not essential to select the most important, and you can focus on different positive displays of affection on different days.

We recommend you identify two types: displays of affection from your parents and displays of affection from other people.

If you want, you can write it down as if it were a diary. That way, you can read them again anytime you want and can remember the major displays of affect that you've received.

The objective of this practice is twofold:

1. Restore a sense of balance and emotional connection with parental figures (if necessary) and with other people (e.g., increase trust in people who have shown us affection).
2. Increase our self-esteem and sense of dignity if it's low. Many people feel unworthy of being loved (especially if they were emotionally deprived as a child).

Remembering the moments you've been loved can improve how you see yourself. If you haven't received affection from someone, it's not because you're unlovable. Other people in your life may not know how to show love because of their history or personality, and this is not your fault.

Remember...

- Before moving towards practices of giving affection to ourselves and to others, it's important to identify and recognize what your attachment pattern is.
- The main difference between the secure pattern and insecure patterns is the relationship you have with yourself and with others.
- Shame is an emotion that we feel when we don't want others to know something about us, since we think that if they do, they will stop loving us or change the way they see us. One way to repair this is with compassion.
- Relationship refers to what we think, what we feel, and how we act, as well as what expectations we have of ourselves and of others.
- Securely attached people can spontaneously give affection (they don't need to be asked), they don't feel bad about giving affection, and they don't feel vulnerable.
- We usually classify people into three categories: friends, enemies, and neutral people. Usually, it is easiest to give affection to friends, somewhat more difficult to give affection to neutral people and, finally, more complicated to give affection to enemies. Keep this in mind when approaching your practice of giving affection to others and start with the easiest, progressing little by little to the hardest.
- Remembering the moments when you have been loved can help you have a better relationship with yourself.

9 Self-Assessment Questions

You're doing great! Now, let's review what you've learned in this module. We'll present you with a series of questions about the most important aspects. Don't worry if you don't know an answer, these questions are designed to help you.

Please answer the following questions:

	True/ False
1. In compassion practices, words are used to develop a critical, demanding, and rigid attitude towards yourself and towards others. This is the best way to strengthen yourself in life and not suffer.	
2. Recognizing and remembering positive and negative aspects of your parents (or main caregivers) is useful to balance and reconcile your relationship with them.	
3. When people feel they haven't been loved, it's because they deserved due to their own personal characteristics.	
4. When carrying out the practices of giving affection to others, it's best to start with friends and, little by little, move towards the neutral people and enemies.	

Explanation of Self-Assessment Questions

Question	Correct answer	Explanation
1. In compassion practices, words are used to develop a critical, demanding, and rigid attitude towards yourself and towards others. This is the best way to strengthen yourself in life and not suffer.	False	Just the opposite! In compassion practices words are used as a way to develop affection and care towards yourself and towards others through words of kindness and affection. This is a very powerful strategy for structuring our internal dialogue, the way we talk to ourselves, so that it's compassionate.
2. Recognizing and remembering positive and negative aspects of your parents (or main caregivers) is useful to balance and reconcile your relationship with them.	True	Exactly. Recognizing and remembering the positive and negative aspects of your parents (or main caregivers) is useful to balance and reconcile your relationship with them. This is a good strategy to adjust expectations, recognizing that it is very difficult for parents (or main caregivers) to have always met your expectations, to have always been fair and affectionate. Furthermore, it's a first step towards reconciling with this key figure which helps you develop a secure attachment pattern.
3. When people feel they haven't been loved, it's because they deserved it due to their own personal characteristics.	False	This is false. The truth is that, if you haven't received affection from someone, it's not because of you but because of the characteristics and circumstances of that person, something that is beyond your own control. A helpful strategy to have a better relationship with yourself in these cases would be to remember moments in your life when you have been loved by someone.
4. When carrying out the practices of giving affection to others, it's best to start with friends and, little by little, move towards the neutral people and enemies.	True	It's generally easier to give affection to friends – people you know well and have an emotional bond with. With practice, you can work on giving affection to the neutral people, and finally, thanks to the work of compassion, you can try the more difficult step of giving affection to enemies. However, the latter is usually worked on in advanced compassion. We recommend starting with friends and neutral people.

10 Homework

Next, we are going to present you with a series of tasks. As you already know, carrying out the tasks that we propose in each module is a fundamental pillar of this program. Remember, the more you know and practice, the more you can benefit from the online intervention. Therefore, in addition to reading, listening, and reviewing all the information that is included in each module, we ask you to put the homework into practice. Think of a toolbox that you go to when you have a problem. We are giving you valuable tools. Now you have to learn how to use them. And don't forget: The more time you put into learning the material and doing the exercises, the more you'll benefit from it.

In this module we ask you to perform the following tasks:

- Read the content of this module carefully, and review all the material it includes.
- Do Formal Practice 1 "Give Affection to Friends and Neutral People" at least once *.
- Do Formal Practice 2 "Giving Ourselves Affection" at least once *.
- Do Formal Practice 3 "Repairing Shame" at least once *.
- Do Formal Practice 4 "Reconciling with Parental Figures" at least once *.
- Complete Exercise 1 "Three Positive and Three Negative Things About Your Parental Figures."
- Do Informal Practice 1 "Greatest Show of Affection Ever Received" several times a day for 2 to 3 days a week.
- Use the Compassion Practice Journal to record your meditative practice on a daily basis.
- Keep practicing the Formal Practice of "Compassionate Breathing" and "Compassionate Body Scan" at least once a week each.
- Review any previous modules that you have questions about.
- Do any task/exercise/meditation that we have recommended and you haven't done yet.

* *Note*: Depending on your situation, we recommend doing the formal practices of this module several times a week on alternate days.

Congratulations! You have finished Module 5 "Working on Ourselves."

In this module you have deepened the importance of affection towards yourself and towards others in order to promote a secure attachment, also changing aspects of the relationship with others and with yourself.

We encourage you to continue practicing everything you have seen in this module. Keep going; you're more than halfway through the intervention!

If you want, you can see the module summary in Annex 5. You can also download the audio of the formal practices of this module.

Annexes of the Module 5

Annex 1. Formal Practice of Giving Affection to Friends and Neutral People

Adopt the meditation posture that you usually use.

Dedicate the first moments to feel your body, the contact of the feet with the ground, and take several deep breaths, slowly letting go of previous thoughts and emotions.

Little by little, bring to mind some person for whom you feel affection, someone you get along well with, and with which you have no conflict. That is, someone with whom you feel close. It might be someone who is a friend, relative, or another person in your life. Stay a few moments selecting that person.

Now, imagine that you are in a room sitting, in meditation, and that person enters the room and sits next to you and also starts to meditate. Because you're friends, you know about that person's history, including moments of suffering and moments of happiness throughout their life.

Focus on the moments of suffering that person has experienced, recognizing that they've suffered just as you've suffered and just as everyone suffers at times. By being aware of their suffering, notice any spontaneous affection that you feel, a natural compassion that you would like to see them free from suffering and enjoying happiness.

Repeat the compassion phrases that best fits for you (e.g., "I hope you can be happy, I hope everything goes well for you, I hope you can achieve peace"). You can use these phrases or others that are appropriate to what you feel or to your way of being. While you say this phrase, you can visualize that you are hugging that person or showing a gesture of affection towards them. You can hug or do any other posture of compassion while imaging how that feeling of affection comes out of you and floods the other person. Repeat these phrases several times, with feeling.

Little by little, imagine that they also feel better, more comforted, by receiving this affection and that you also feel more connected to them. Savor and enjoy that feeling of connection with the other person. Keep in image of the compassionate gesture and the feeling of compassion towards the other person as long as you want. Notice any commitment you feel to express your affection towards the other person and your loved ones when you see them. Little by little, let the image disappear and return to your breath, letting go of the emotions and thoughts that you experienced.

Next, select a person who is completely neutral to you. It may be someone who lives far away, and therefore, you don't know them very well. It can also be a coworker, neighbor, or someone you have seen physically but with whom you don't interact with often, and so you don't really know them.

Once you have selected the person who is neutral to you, imagine that you're in a room sitting, meditating, and that the person enters the room and sits down by your side, to also meditate. Although you don't know them at all, and you don't know about their history; you can imagine that they've had moments of suffering and joy like you and like all of us. When becoming aware of their suffering, notice whether you a spontaneous feeling of affection arises in you, a natural compassion to wish to see them free from suffering and enjoying happiness. Whether or not you feel this, depending on how you feel it, you can repeat in your mind the phrases of compassion that feel the most appropriate (e.g., "I hope you can be happy, I hope everything goes well for you, I hope may you achieve peace"). You can repeat these phrases several times and notice if you can feel that feeling of affection, if you can visualize and even make a compassionate gesture towards them, or if it is complicated by the fact that this is a neutral person. Without forcing yourself, express your affection towards them as you feel it.

Little by little, imagine that this person feels better, more comforted, receiving this affection. Notice how you feel, and whether you've been able to feel connected to this human, even if you don't know them or if it's been harder for you to feel affection for them. Notice this with curiosity, with acceptance, without judging yourself. Observe the difficulties that you may have had generating those feelings of affection, compassion, and try to analyze the reason why. Notice what thoughts appear, what happens. Stay a few seconds observing this.

Stay in the visualization, the compassionate gesture, and the feeling of compassion towards the other person, for as long as you want, noticing any commitment you feel to express your affection towards unknown people when you get the chance. Little by little, let the image disappear and return to your breath, letting go of the emotions and thoughts that you've experienced during the practice, ending it whenever you're ready.

Annex 2. Formal Practice of Giving Ourselves Affection

Begin by adopting the meditation posture that you usually use. Take a few moments to feel your body, the contact with floor, and your posture, and take several deep breaths, letting go of any previous emotions and thoughts.

Gradually, try to visualize yourself, when you were little, specifically when you were a young child. You may not remember when you were 2–3 years old, but you can think of old pictures or stories of yourself that you've seen or heard. Based on this information and the memories you have, imagine the first few years of your childhood and how you were growing. Focus on times of joy and happiness but also on times of sadness and loneliness.

Focus for a minute on those first 10 years of your life, which have been so important in determining who you are and how you understand the world. When you remember your life, the positive and negative experiences you had as a child, you can start to understand how your history has shaped the person you are today.

Then the years went by and you turned 15, 20, or maybe 25 years old. During that period, you might have finished school, started working, or had or did not have sexual relationships and partnerships. Again, focus on both, the negative experiences, the sadness, and the positive experiences, the joys you had.

Inevitably, you got older until you reached your current age. From the perspective of your current age, notice the main moments of sadness, of suffering, that you've had in your life and also the moments of happiness. You can see that you, like all living beings, have tried to find happiness and have tried to avoid suffering. However, despite your best efforts, at times you've experienced suffering. Take a few moments to look at the situations where you tried to be happy and make things to be better but instead experienced greater suffering. This can help you understand other people because this same thing has happened to all of us. In the search for happiness and to avoid suffering, many times, we have instead found more suffering.

Now, at your current age, with the perspective that you have, you can observe the entire life you've lived so far. Take a few moments to give yourself all the affection that you can. Recognize the ways that you deserve affection, because you have tried hard to be happy and make others happy, even if you haven't always achieved it. You can do the compassionate gesture that you prefer (e.g., hugging, touching hands, face, etc.), to feel how you transmit this love and this affection to yourself. Notice whether this is something you do frequently or very rarely.

Stay a few seconds feeling how you merge with this compassionate gesture. Savor and enjoy that sense of connection with yourself, that feeling of gratitude, of well-being, a feeling that connects you with all humanity. You can stay in that posture and with that feeling as long as you would like. When ready, you can turn your attention to your body and to your breath, letting go the emotions and thoughts that you experienced during this practice. Little by little, to finish the exercise, move your body, becoming aware of the room or the place where you are and finishing the practice with a commitment to give affection to yourself, whenever you can, and often, because you deserve it.

Annex 3. Formal Practice of Repairing Shame

Begin the practice by adopting your usual meditation posture. Take some conscious breaths, and feel your body as a whole and keep breathing in and out, consciously.

Little by little, bring to mind any kind of negative beliefs you have about yourself and of which you are ashamed. Let this belief appear freely in your mind, and see how you feel it in your body and how it makes you feel when you think about it.

Shame is an emotion that arises when we do not want others to know something about us, because we think that if they knew, they would stop loving us, or it would change the way they see us.

Recognize and identify what your main shame is. It may be that you consider yourself unintelligent, uneducated, insecure, clumsy, etc. Become aware of in what moments of your life have you felt or others have made you feel that way? And ask yourself: Where does that shame come from? What belief brings that shame to life? Can I learn something from it? Who really cares about this shame?

Almost everyone has felt this way at some point, ashamed and undervalued for very similar personal characteristics or qualities as those you identified. You are not alone in your shame. This emotion arises naturally and from the desire to comply with certain standards of social desirability. Like everyone else, you also want to feel valued, immensely loved, and accepted. But you can allow yourself to accept the parts of yourself that make you feel more vulnerable. Admitting this vulnerability does not make you weak; it makes you stronger.

Now, place your hand on the area of the body where you feel your shame. It can be on your heart or anywhere it creates tension in your body. Stroke it this part of yourself, and direct your breath to that area of your body, healing the wound that shame created. Stay like this for as long as you consider necessary. And whenever you're ready, become aware of your surroundings and start moving your body, ending the practice.

Annex 4. Formal Practice "Reconciliation with Parental Figures"

This exercise may produce intense emotion. If you feel overwhelmed during the exercise, direct your attention to your breath, or focus on where you feel the emotion in. your body. This will help you disengage from the practice. You can also end the practice at any point.

First, take the meditation posture that you usually use. Notice your body posture, the contact of your feet with the ground, and take several deep breaths to calm yourself, letting go of any previous emotions and thoughts.

Little by little, begin to feel, on your right, the presence of one of your parental figures. This may be your mother or father or someone else who raised you. Imagine them at the age they were when you were little. Imagine this regardless of whether they are currently alive or not. Feel that they are there with you physically, not just as an image but in the room with you.

Based on what you know about them, imagine them throughout their lifespan. Start when they were a little child. Although you didn't know them at that age, you may have seen pictures of them when they were a child. Imagine them developing as a child, little by little, across the first 5 to 10 years of their life. Consider what their life was like at that point, what their environment was like.

Think about any negative situations that this parental figure experienced. And also think about the positive experiences, the joys. You are seeing their history: what they experienced and the things that happened to them. Try to understand how was this person's childhood, the moments of sadness and suffering, and all their experiences combined were shaping their character.

Little by little, imagine the person getting older, turning ages 10, 15, and 20 years old. Notice how their physical appearance and environment change, and think about any negative or joyful experiences they had over these years. Try to understand how all this shaped the type of parental figure they became.

Continue to observe the years go by, as the person turns ages 30, 35, and 40 years old. Remember the age they were when you were born and when your siblings, if you have any, were born. Observe how this person was getting older as you grew up. Remember the positive and negative situations that were happening to them and to your family at the time of your childhood, all the way up until their current age or until they passed away.

Try to identify with the life of this person, live it as if you were them, especially the moments of suffering, as if you were the one who had lived it. At the same time, see if you can feel any affection for them during the times that they were suffering. This person, like you, like all living beings, was struggling to achieve happiness and avoid suffering. See if you can empathize with their genuine efforts. Recognize that, many times, all that effort didn't end in happiness but in suffering.

Now think of some times throughout your life where you had differences, anger, criticism, or difficulties with this person. Try to remember the bad times that you experienced with them. Now remember any good moments you had with them. If it feels comfortable to you see if you can feel embraced by this parental figure, at whatever age you want (when you were little or currently). Consider the possibility that, despite their mistakes and the suffering they may have caused you, they may have been doing the best they were able to. And like most of us humans, in their struggle to achieve happiness, they sometimes found even more suffering. If it feels comfortable to you, hug this parental figure for a few seconds, and thank them for any good they've given you. If you don't feel comfortable doing so, that is also ok.

At a pace that feels comfortable for you, return to viewing the parental figure at your right side. Turn your attention to your breath, observe any emotions that emerged, and create a space of calm for yourself.

If you do not have another parental figure, finish the practice, giving thanks for anything good you received from this parental figure as well as other people throughout your life. Stay a few moments with this feeling of gratitude that connects you with all humanity. When you're ready, slowly, return with full attention to your breathing, letting go of any thoughts and emotions you felt, and slowly; when you're done, begin to move your body, opening your eyes, and ending the practice.

If you have another parental figure who is different from the person you thought about before, continue the practice. Imagine that this other parental figure is sitting at your left side. Again, feel that they are there with you physically, not just as an image but in the room with you.

Based on what you know about them, imagine them throughout their lifespan. Start when they were a little child. Although you didn't know them at that age, you may have seen pictures of them when they were a child. Imagine them developing as a child, little by little, across the first 5 to 10 years of their life. Consider what their life was like at that point, what their environment was like.

Think about any negative situations that this parental figure experienced. And also think about the positive experiences, the joys. You are seeing their history: what they experienced and the things that happened to them. Try to understand how was this person's childhood, the moments of sadness and suffering, and all their experiences combined were shaping their character.

Little by little, imagine the person getting older, turning ages 10, 15, and 20 years old. Notice how their physical appearance and environment change, and think about any negative or joyful experiences they had over these years. Try to understand how all this shaped the type of parental figure they became.

Continue to observe the years go by, as the person turns ages 30, 35, and 40 years old. Remember the age they were when you were born and when your siblings, if you have any, were born. Observe how this person was getting older as you grew up. Remember the positive and negative situations that were happening to them and to your family at the time of your childhood, all the way up until their current age or until they passed away.

Try to identify with the life of this person, live it as if you were them, especially the moments of suffering, as if you were the one who had lived it. At the same time, see if you can feel any affection for them during the times that they were suffering. This person, like you, like all living beings, was struggling to achieve happiness and avoid suffering. See if you can empathize with their genuine efforts. Recognize that, many times, all that effort didn't end in happiness but in suffering.

Now think of some times throughout your life where you had differences, anger, criticism, or difficulties with this person. Try to remember the bad times that you experienced with them. Now remember any good moments you had with them. If it feels comfortable to you see if you can feel embraced by this parental figure, at whatever age you want (when you were little or currently). Consider the possibility that, despite their mistakes and the suffering they may have caused you, they may have been doing best they were able to. And like most of us humans, in their struggle to achieve happiness, they sometimes found even more suffering. If it feels comfortable to you, you can hug this parental figure for a few seconds if you'd like. However, if you don't feel comfortable hugging, that's ok too. Thank them for any good they've given you and see if you can genuinely forgive any suffering they caused you.

If it feels comfortable, imagine that you, your two parental figures, and any other people who are important in your life (partner, children, or some very significant friend, other relatives) all embrace. Imagine this even if they are no longer living. Allow yourself to savor and enjoy that feeling of connection with all of them, that feeling of affection. Become aware that all the people of this world, including your parental figures, partner, and relatives, have tried to escape from suffering and search for happiness. However, recognize that we all have often created a chain of suffering that includes us, our loved ones, and many other people. This has happened to all humans, generating a web of pain that connects all human beings. Realizing this can help you understand and reconcile with the harm you received from your parental figures and from other people in this world. You can also forgive yourself for the suffering you have caused.

Give thanks for any good you have received from your parental figures and other people throughout your life. Stay a few moments with this feeling of gratitude that connects you with all humanity. Slowly, return, with full attention to your breathing, letting go of any thoughts and emotions. Slowly, when you are ready, begin to move your body, opening your eyes, and ending the practice.

Annex 5. Summary of the Module

Objectives of the Module

- Understand the importance of affection (or compassion) towards yourself and towards others, and learn how this will help you create a secure attachment pattern.
- Do the Formal Practice "Giving Affection to Friends and Neutral People."
- Do the Formal Practice "Giving Ourselves Affection."
- Learn the causes of shame and to learn how to handle this difficult emotion.

- Do the Formal Practice "Reconciliation with Parental Figures," and reflect on the difficulties and different emotions with the practice.
- Identify Three Positive and Three Negative Things About Your Parental Figure(s) through a practical exercise, to continue reflecting on the relationship you've had with them.
- Do Informal Practice 1 "The Greatest Show of Affection Ever Received."
- Reflect on how we usually classify people into three categories: friends, enemies, and neutral people.

Module Contents

Importance of Affection Towards Ourselves and Towards Others Before moving towards practices of giving affection towards yourselves and towards others, it's important to identify and recognize what your attachment pattern is.

The main difference between secure and insecure attachment patterns is the relationship you established with yourself and with others. By relationship we mean: what we think, what we feel, how we act, and what expectations we have of ourselves and of others.

It is very important that your internal dialogue is compassionate; therefore, we use kind and compassionate words to express affection for yourself and for others.

Formal Practice 1: Give Affection to Friends and Neutral People We encourage you to work on expressing affection towards friends, which is usually easy and spontaneous, versus neutral people and enemies, which is something that's more complicated. After the practice, we recommend reflecting on any difficulties you experienced doing the exercise.

Securely attached people can give affection spontaneously, they don't feel bad for giving affection, and don't feel vulnerable.

Formal Practice 2: Giving Yourself Affection Once you've been able to give affection to people you already love and who are neutral to you, you can move on to giving yourself affection.

For most people it's more difficult to give affection to themselves than giving it to others. After the practice, we recommend you reflect for a moment on the difficulties you have giving yourself affection. *Remember: You can be a good attachment figure to yourself (although not necessarily the only one).*

Shame Shame is an emotion that we feel when we don't want others to know something about us because we think that if they knew, they'd stop loving us or would change the way they see us. One way to work on this emotion is with compassion, through the Formal Practice 3 *Repairing Shame.*

Formal Practice 4: Reconciliation with Parental Figures Parental figures or early caregivers are the key figures in the development of our attachment patterns. Reconciling with Parental Figures, whether in real life or not, could be a very healing practice in compassion-based intervention. If you don't feel ready to do this, that's ok too.

Homework

- Read the content of this module carefully and review all the material it includes.
- Do Formal Practice 1 "Give Affection to Friends and Neutral People" at least once *.
- Do Formal Practice 2 "Giving Ourselves Affection" at least once *.
- Do Formal Practice 3 "Repairing Shame" at least once *.
- Do Formal Practice 4 "Reconciling with Parental Figures" at least once *.
- Complete Exercise 1 "Three Positive and Three Negative Things About Your Parental Figures."
- Do Informal Practice 1 "Greatest Show of Affection Ever Received" several times a day for 2–3 days a week.
- Use the Compassion Practice Journal to record your meditative practice on a daily basis.
- Keep practicing the Formal Practice of "Compassionate Breathing" and "Compassionate Body Scan" at least once a week each.
- Review any previous modules that you have questions about.
- Do any task/exercise/meditation that we have recommended and you haven't done yet.

Depending on your situation, we recommend doing the *formal practices* of this module several times a week on alternate days.

Chapter 8
Module 6: Understanding the Importance of Forgiveness

Module Objectives

In this module, we want to help you achieve the following goals:

- Deepen your understanding of what forgiveness is.
- Understand the concept of forgiveness and its phases.
- Learn how to structure the practice of forgiveness.
- Reflect on the importance and the usefulness of forgiveness to yourself and to others.
- Practice forgiveness toward yourself and toward others.
- Understand the things that can make it hard to forgive.
- Learn the main resources to help you forgive.
- Understand the suffering of others and give them affection, so you can start to do it in everyday life.

Go ahead with the module. Don't feel like you need to hurry through it. It's more important to try to understand all the concepts that are presented and practice the exercises.

Module Contents

1. The Concept of Forgiveness
2. Forgiveness and Justice
3. The Usefulness of Forgiveness
4. Phases of Forgiveness
5. How to Structure the Practice of Forgiveness
6. Formal Practice 1: Forgiving Yourself
7. Formal practice 2: Asking Others for Forgiveness
8. Formal Practice 3: Forgiving Others and Giving Compassion to Enemies
9. Resources to Use to Generate Forgiveness

Supplementary Information The online version contains supplementary material available at https://doi.org/10.1007/978-3-031-38032-7_8.

J. García-Campayo et al., *The Attachment-Based Compassion Therapy*,
https://doi.org/10.1007/978-3-031-38032-7_8

10. Recapitulation
11. Informal Practice 1: Interdependence
12. Informal Practice 2: Compassion in Daily Life
13. Self-Assessment Questions
14. Homework
15. Annexes of the Module

In this module you will learn about the concept of forgiveness, the things that can make it hard to forgive, the importance of forgiveness toward yourself and others, and the main resources you can use to forgive. The goal is to be more compassionate toward yourself and toward others, paving the way to be compassionate toward your enemies. In addition, informal practice will help you understand the suffering of others and give them affection, making it easier to apply it in your daily life.

1 The Concept of Forgiveness

Definitions of Forgiveness

Forgiveness is often defined as "an individual, voluntary internal process of letting go of feelings and thoughts of resentment, bitterness, anger, and the need for vengeance and retribution toward someone who we believe has wronged us, including ourselves" (https://positivepsychology.com/forgiveness-benefits/).

The word "forgive" comes from the Latin word "perdonare," meaning "to give completely, without reservation." This means that the person who was hurt gives to the person who hurt them a gift by pardoning the injury.

While there are many definitions of forgiveness, the following three components are generally emphasized:

- Behavioral/Decision-Based Forgiveness: Forgiving is something that we choose to do based on our own will power (DiBlasio, 1998).
- Cognitive Forgiveness: Forgiving requires changing how we think about the event that hurt us. It involves recognizing that there are factors that are beyond anyone's control/fault (Gordon et al., 2005).
- Emotional Forgiveness: Forgiving means letting go of anger, resentment and vengefulness, and shifting to emotions of compassion (Worthington, 2006).

Some believe that all three aspects of forgiveness (e.g., behavioral, cognitive, and emotional) need to change for a person to fully forgive.

However, in this intervention we take the approach that the process of forgiveness can take many forms. It may involve acceptance and empathy, as well as engaging in perspective-taking and benefit-finding.

Your understanding of forgiveness may be influenced by your upbringing, religion, or culture. For example, in Christianity forgiveness is considered the highest display of love and a defining attribute of what it means to be a good Christian.

A common challenge that many individuals face with forgiveness is that many have been raised based on their family backgrounds or religions to view forgiveness as an "obligation."

In this intervention, we view forgiveness as a choice rather than an obligation. Moreover, forgiveness often takes time. Usually, we need to allow ourselves to feel anger, hurt, and grief before we can forgive.

What Forgiveness Is not

Forgiveness is not:

- Pardoning
- Condoning
- Excusing an offense
- Forgetting about the offense
- Reconciliation (this could occur as part of the forgiveness process but is not necessary/relevant for everyone's forgiveness process)

Forgiveness is not pardoning, condoning, or excusing an offense or forgetting about it. It is also not the same as reconciliation although that can occur as part of the forgiveness process. Forgiveness is a progressive process, not something that happens immediately. Forgiving is not an obligation, but something you do voluntarily.

We provide additional information about what forgiveness is *not* and clarifies how forgiveness can be healthy for us personally.

- *Forgiveness does not imply that justice is not done*: If the individual who has done harm has committed a crime, there should be justice, and the person shouldn't be exempt. If this didn't happen, it would reinforce crime in society and would suggest that crime has no consequences. Forgiveness is basically an internal act, which benefits the victim and helps the victim end any ruminations of hatred/victimhood for the event that occurred.
- These loops of thought can affect our entire lives and prevent us from enjoying the present moment. Feelings of hatred can take a big toll on our mental and physical health.
- Forgiveness allows us to get closure on a difficult period in our lives. Otherwise, we may be caught for the rest of our lives on the suffering with a negative event.
- *Forgiveness is not denying harm*: Denial is one of the most common ways of coping, and it's often used by children. However, recognizing the damage that was done and the pain you feel is necessary to start the process of healing and forgiving. Recognizing this might start with saying to yourself: "They have hurt me and this hurts."

- *Forgiveness does not imply forgetting*: Sometimes our mind unconsciously forgets painful events as a way to cope. However, the trauma will come out at some point and in some form (e.g., as physical symptoms, phobias, etc.). Forgiveness doesn't mean forgetting. It means successfully overcoming the trauma so that you can reduce any negative consequences it might have on the rest of your life.
- *Forgiving is not an immediate process* but a progressive one: When two children fight, adults usually tell them to forgive each other. But forgiveness is not something we can force or do immediately after someone has hurt us. Forgiveness requires time to grieve any feeling of loss, validate the anger you might feel, recognize the sense of injustice, and build your resilience. It's a healing process (and sometimes only achieved through therapy), which can take weeks to years, if at all.
- *Forgiveness is not an obligation, but should be your choice*: The idea of forgiveness as mandatory is often linked to specific religions. However, for the purpose of this compassion-based intervention, we view forgiveness as something you choose to do, not something you have to do.
- *Forgiving does not imply reconciliation*: Forgiveness does not imply that you have a relationship with that person again. In fact, in cases of abuse or bullying, we recommend that you don't have contact with the person who hurt you. Forgiveness is something that happens internally, and it's not necessary to have contact with the perpetrator.

2 Forgiveness and Justice

Humans view relationships as reciprocal. In other words, there's a give-and-take to the relationship.

If we do something positive for someone, we expect that person to reciprocate and do something positive for us at some point (not necessarily right away but at some point in the future) and in some way (not necessarily with the same intensity but in some proportion). In fact, relationships often depend on this give-and-take. If there's not a minimum level of reciprocity, the relationship will tend to break.

When one person hurts another person, it breaks the give-and-take in a relationship. For the hurt person to continue the relationship, it usually requires some sort of repair or compensation by the person who caused the harm. If not, the hurt person feels a sense of injustice.

Perceived injustice, that is, the feeling that one has been harmed and does not obtain some form of compensation, is associated with a worse prognosis of the disease and greater suffering. Examples would include people who have suffered traffic or work accidents they perceive to not be their fault or in patients affected with chronic diseases and who feel mistreated by the health system. If we consider equal severity of an injury, the person who experiences perceived injustice will be worse off than if the person themselves were responsible for the damage.

Examples of common reactions to perceived injustice are seeking revenge, redirecting of anger to others, and continued feelings of hatred and resentment toward perpetrators.

Forgiveness is one option when someone harms us. But there are also alternatives to forgiveness as listed here:

- Revenge: Throughout history, people, society, and civilizations many have sought revenge. Laws reflect this. For example, ancient Egypt and Jewish culture had the rule that a person receive the same punishment that they inflicted on someone else. This is described in the famous quote, "An eye for an eye and a tooth for a tooth."[1, 2] Germanic people called this blood revenge (i.e., "bultrache"), and, even today, many Muslim countries maintain a similar principle based on Islamic or Sharia law.
- Displacement of Violence: Sometimes revenge isn't possible, not for lack of desire but because the aggressor has more power than the victim. In these cases, some people who have been victims repeat the cycle of violence with other people. This is common in gender violence. For example, a person may watch their father act in a violent way toward their mother or experience violence directly from their father. This person may then go on to act in the same violent way toward their partner or children. This can also be seen in bullying at school or "mobbing," which is a form of group bullying in the workplace (García-Campayo et al., 2004). A victim of bullying or mobbing may bully other school children or engage in mobbing with other co-workers or family members.
- Hate Maintained: In many cases, the person doesn't seek revenge or redirect violence toward others. If the person doesn't forgive, this often means continuing to feel hatred or resentment toward the person who caused harm. Sometimes people hold out hope for compensation in the future (in the case of religion, in the afterlife) or through justice. However, if a person continues to feel hatred, it can make them chronically stressed. This can lead to other physical and psychological illnesses.

In general, these alternatives to forgiveness may be attempts to restructure perceived injustice. While it may seem effective in the short term, in the long term these strategies often maintain and increase suffering as well as prevent giving compassion toward oneself and toward others (García-Campayo et al., 2016a, b).

3 The Usefulness of Forgiveness

Forgiveness is a very useful response both on a social and individual level.

[1] Code of Hammurabi; Law of the Talion from the Latin "talis" or "tale," meaning "similar."

[2] Exodus 21: 23–25 and Leviticus 24: 18–20p.

(a) *At the social level*: Forgiveness is useful since people often experience conflicts (e.g., work disagreements, divorce proceedings, owing money, etc.). Society relies on justice, but forgiveness is important too. Without forgiveness, it would be difficult to have social cohesion and collective goals.
(b) *At the individual level*: Long-lasting hatred or hostility produces chronic stress which produces persistently high cortisol in the blood. These persistently high cortisol levels activate inflammation. This process is at the basis of a large number of psychiatric and somatic illnesses.

In sum, we should try to develop forgiveness, not just for ethical or spiritual reasons but also because chronic resentment is bad for our physical and mental health.

4 Phases of Forgiveness

There are four stages of forgiveness to reach acceptance:

1. Recognition: Becoming aware of the harm that was done, without denying or minimizing it. Experiencing all the suffering associated with it.
2. Responsibility: Assuming responsibility (if applicable) for the part we played in contributing to the event that caused damage.
3. Expression: Openly expressing emotions (e.g., anger, sadness, hurt, fear) and not just ruminating about them. Experiencing these emotions with understanding, affection, kindness, and non-judgment. That is, with compassion.
4. Recreation: Developing a new way of understanding yourself in relation to the person who caused you harm. The person who caused harm may be you or it may be someone else. This final stage usually brings a new sense of life that integrates everything you learned during the acceptance process (Fig. 8.1).

5 How to Structure the Practice of Forgiveness

We recommend structuring the practice of forgiveness in the following order:

- Forgiving yourself
- Asking others for forgiveness
- Forgiving others and give compassion to enemies
- Forgiving loved ones who have harmed us

In this module, we will focus on forgiving yourself (Formal Practice 1), asking other for forgiveness (Formal Practice 2), and forgiving others and giving compassion to enemies (Formal Practice 3).

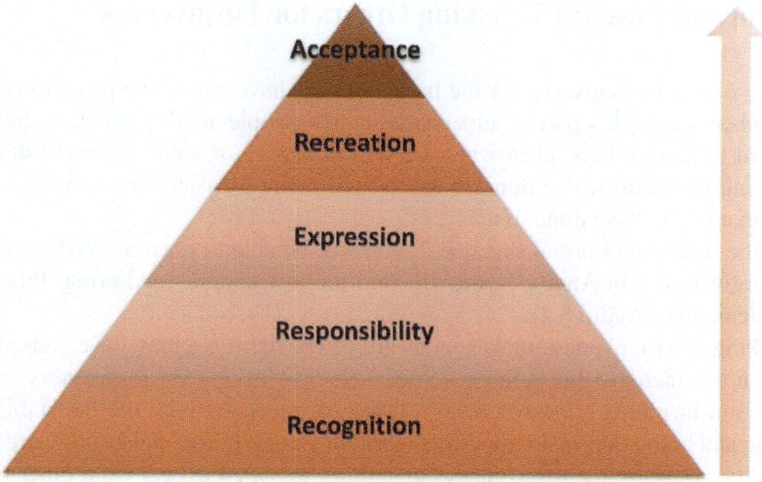

Fig. 8.1 Stages of forgiveness to reach acceptance

6 Formal Practice 1: Forgiving Yourself

We tend to treat others the way we treat ourselves. If we're affectionate toward ourselves, it's easier for us to be affectionate with other people. On the other hand, if we're demanding and unforgiving of ourselves, it is almost impossible for us to give affection and forgive others. Feelings of guilt (the main cause of chronic depression and grief), shame, and self- criticism are related to not forgiving yourself and being self-demanding and self-critical.

Forgiving yourself for the mistakes you may have made throughout your life is a very healthy practice psychologically.

You can do the Practice of Forgiving Yourself with the audio below. In Annex 1 you can also read the transcript for the Practice of Forgiving Yourself (Supplementary Audio 8.1).

Generally, it will be necessary to repeat this practice several times in order to generate the feeling of forgiveness and well-being, as well as review the different situations in life in which we have hurt ourselves in some way. Sometimes it is possible to forgive yourself for a specific situation but not for others, so it is necessary to review the main situations and be able to forgive yourself for all of them.

We encourage you to review the different situations, at your own pace, and progress as you feel ready.

7 Formal Practice 2: Asking Others for Forgiveness

Asking others to forgive us for the harm we may have caused helps us to connect with other people. It's part of understanding that people aren't perfect. As humans, we tend to harm others, even when we don't mean to or aren't aware of doing it. Realizing the harm we've done to others will make it easier for us to forgive the harm that others have done to us.

In the following Formal Practice 2, you will be able to practice "Asking Others for Forgiveness." In Annex 2 you will find the instructions for Formal Practice 2 (Supplementary Audio 8.2).

Asking for forgiveness makes us aware of the harm we may have caused. The goal isn't to increase our guilt but to decrease it by asking for forgiveness (even if the person has already passed away). It also connects us with the inevitability of hurting and being hurt in an imperfect world like ours. It also makes us aware of the difficulty in asking for forgiveness (something we often expect from other people who have harmed us).

8 Formal Practice 3: Forgiving Others and Giving Compassion to Enemies

We can have strong feelings toward people who have hurt us or who we consider enemies. In these cases, it's difficult to give affection or compassion to these people. A helpful first step is to try to forgive them. This may not be possible, but it can be very healing for you personally if you're open to it. Later, if you're ready, you can also practice compassion.

If you're, you can try the practice of forgiving others and giving compassion to enemies through the following audio. When doing the exercise, only focus on the people who you feel capable of forgiving at this time. It's ok if you're not ready to do this exercise. You can skip it for now and you can always go back to it later (Supplementary Audio 8.3).

You'll also find the instructions for the practice in Annex 3.

9 Resources to Use to Generate Forgiveness

The main resources to generate forgiveness are:

- Recognizing the limited freedom in human behavior.
- Dealing with perceived injustice.
- Healthy reperception.

Recognizing the Limited Freedom in Human Behavior

Thinking that another person hurt us on purpose can make us feel especially bad. We may feel hate or resentment toward that person. If we were hurt because of natural causes (e.g., an accident due to a falling rock), the negative event doesn't impact us as much psychologically.

When we think that we would act very differently (and better) than the person who hurt us, it can help to recognize that we may have done the same thing if we were in that person's shoes. What saves us from that behavior (and from that outcome) is having a different history and life story.

This equation summarizes the causes of human behavior:

> Behavior = Genetics + Physiology + Learning History + Situation

In other words, we can recognize that other people do things because of who they are, because they may not be able to act otherwise. Remembering this can help us feel better about situations where we were hurt. It helps us to not take it as personally and to see that people are victims of themselves.

Dealing with Perceived Injustice

When another person harms us, we expect them to receive a fair punishment. If the act goes unpunished or we feel the punishment is insufficient, we might develop a feeling of hostility and discontent with the world, in other words, perceived injustice.

Religions solve this by saying that human justice is imperfect and that God will judge that person in the afterlife (in theistic religions) or that karma will give the person what they deserve (in Hinduism and Buddhism).

If you don't have religious beliefs, you can view perceived injustice in the following ways:

- Because the person who harmed you will likely treat others the same way, they will likely receive negative consequences from society for their actions. We can have compassion on them for the negative consequences they may face in the future.
- The idea that the world has to be fair is a misconception. The world is the way it is: it's not fair for lions to eat zebras or for a child to die of cancer, and yet these things happen. This means that it's irrational to expect the world to be fair.

Healthy Reperception

This is one of the most effective therapeutic techniques when negative events happen to us. It consists of not focusing on the negative aspects associated with the event (not over-identifying with them), which we tend to get attached, but rather focusing on the positive aspects that this situation has been able to generate. These positive aspects, even in the most adverse situation (e.g., the death of a child), are always of two types:

(a) *Learning and Resilience*: If I have been able to overcome/survive/adapt to a situation as negative as this, I can face any other situation in life, because it will likely not be as adverse as this one. In other words, it's made me stronger.
(b) *Help Others*: What I have learned throughout this process can help other people in my situation. I can feel useful knowing that my experience has helped other people to not suffer so much. Therefore, I can give meaning to my suffering by helping to reduce the suffering of others.

10 Recapitulation

Recapitulation is the act of retracing or re-experiencing your life so far (Castaneda, 2001, 2011). In this case, we want you to focus on your closest relationships during different periods of your life. This practice is tied to forgiveness because we often experience hurt in our close relationships (either they have hurt us or we have hurt them), and we may have unresolved issues.

> The purpose of this practice is to re-experience your life during specific periods of time. Remember your life in chunks of 5 years and go in consecutive order (e.g., age 0–5, age 6–10, age 11–15, etc.). For each period of 5 years, recall your closest relationships during that time.

By following these instructions, you can practice forgiving those who have hurt you. You can work on forgiving them for the damage done to you and to others. If you do this enough times, eventually you will have "recovered" all the emotional energy linked to these conflicts.

This practice is optional, and we recommend doing it at your own pace, once you feel that you have worked through the previous practices of forgiveness.

11 Informal Practice 1: Interdependence

Interdependence means knowing that everything (e.g., objects, living things, circumstances) that happens in this world is the result of causes and consequences related and dependent on each other. Nothing happens independently and in isolation.

There are two things to consider when doing this informal practice:

(a) With external objects: This is when you reflect on all the relationships, causes, conditions, and consequences necessary for that object to be with you.

For example, when we are eating a food (e.g., a raisin), we could become aware and reflect on the contribution of the land where it was grown, the water that has watered it, the sun that has made it mature, etc., as well as many people (the seller, the transporter, the farmer) and the wisdom of humanity for centuries that the art of agriculture has transmitted.

This reasoning with all objects leads us to be aware of interdependence and, consequently, to thank the world and many people for what we have.

(b) With ourselves: Every time we feel too proud of something and think that "we" have achieved what we have, we can reflect that everything we are is due to many people who have helped us in our lives and have made us who we are (parents, family and friends, partners, teachers, etc.). If we are what we are, it is not only because of our own merits but because of what many people have done for us throughout our lives, and, likely, we have not been able to thank enough.

With this informal practice, we realize how much we owe to other people throughout our lives. We will also be aware that we haven't been able to fully return the favor for the people who have helped us. Others, we couldn't even thank because we're no longer in contact with them. But there's always a way to "repay" what they've done for us: by doing something for humanity, for other people who will likely never be able to return the favor, etc. In this way, with this kind of chain of favors, we give back to the world part of what we have received from it.

12 Informal Practice: Compassion in Daily Life

Informal compassion practices are a way of using compassion in daily life. It can produce greater changes in the individual than formal practices, but we often need the base of formal practices first. We recommend incorporating these practices, progressively, into your daily routine.

Here are some practices that can be done in daily life to reinforce acceptance and compassion:

1. *Acceptance*

    (a) Don't criticize yourself, see the good in you. When you identify a thought, emotion, or behavior that you don't like, don't criticize yourself globally (e.g., "I'm stupid, how can I think this?"). View the thought objectively and send compassion to yourself. You are that emotion or thought, but not only that, you're also other healthy emotions and thoughts. If you prefer, you can do this instead: You are not that emotion or thought that has appeared in your mind, since those things are always changing, but your core self transcends those difficult aspects that may appear in you. Therefore, look for the good in yourself.

    (b) Don't criticize other people; see the good in them. Do to others as you would do to yourself. You won't be able to be compassionate with yourself if you aren't compassionate with others and vice versa. If you have something to say to that person, say so, but don't criticize them in front of others. You can think of the positive aspects of that person. You can also develop empathy for that person by thinking: "If I had the same circumstances as that person, I might be doing the same thing."

2. *Compassion*

    (a) Practice compassion while walking. Throughout the day we can give compassion to the people we see every day. Each day we can select one or two people we meet on the street or at work. We can visualize ourselves sending affection and repeating compassionate phrases toward them. This informal practice lasts about 1–2 min and can be done at any time of the day (walking on the street, on breaks at work, etc.).

    (b) Be aware of compassion in people around you: We likely receive compassion from others on a regular basis (e.g., they ask about our families, offer us a smile, etc.). Be aware of the kindness that other people show you, let yourself be happy about it, and appreciate it.

    (c) Do an act of generosity every day: We can show affection and compassion to people around us: a smile, a detail, a word of thanks, etc. You can try to increase the happiness in the world by starting with your environment. If we, as people who practice compassion, don't help the world get a little bit better, who will?

Remember...

Forgiveness is often defined as "an individual, voluntary internal process of letting go of feelings and thoughts of resentment, bitterness, anger, and the need for vengeance and retribution toward someone who we believe has wronged us, including ourselves" (https://positivepsychology.com/forgiveness-benefits/).

- Human beings base interpersonal relationships on reciprocity. Generating harm to another person breaks reciprocity and demands reparation.
- Less useful alternatives to forgiveness when damage is generated are: revenge, redirection of violence, and sustained hatred.

- Forgiveness is a very useful behavior both at a social level (improves relationships and cohesion) and at an individual level helps with diseases associated with chronic stress produced by sustained hatred).
- The phases from forgiveness to acceptance are (1) recognition, (2) responsibility, (3) expression, and (4) recreation.
- Forgiveness does mean lack of justice or forgetting or denying the damage. Forgiveness is a voluntary, progressive process that does not require reconciliation with the other person.
- We recommend structuring the practice of forgiveness in the following order: (1) Forgive yourself, (2) ask others for forgiveness, (3) forgive others and give compassion to enemies, and (4) forgive loved ones who have harmed us.
- The most useful mechanisms to develop forgiveness are as follows: the recognition of the limited freedom in the conduct of human beings and the handling of perceived injustice and healthy reperceptions.

13 Self-Assessment Questions

You're doing great. Now, let's review what you have learned in this module. For this, we will present you with a series of questions about the most important aspects. Don't worry if you don't know an answer; these questions are designed to help you.

Please answer the following questions:

Question	True	False
1. Forgiveness is a very useful behavior both personally and socially.	T	F
2. Forgiveness involves lack of justice, forgetting, and denying the harm.	T	F
3. To begin with the practice of forgiveness, it is recommended to start with the enemies or people who have hurt us.	T	F
4. Healthy reperception is one of the most effective therapeutic mechanisms for negative events.	T	F

Explanation of Self-Assessment Questions

Question	Correct answer	Explanation
1. Forgiveness is a very useful behavior both personally and socially.	True	You got it right. At the social level, it helps to improve relationships and social cohesion. On an individual level, it helps reduce resentment/hatred which, in turn, reduces associated chronic stress.
2. Forgiveness involves a lack of justice, forgetting, and denying the harm.	False	Forgiveness does not imply forgetting or denying the harm or that there won't be justice Forgiveness is a voluntary, progressive process that does not require reconciliation with the other person.

Question	Correct answer	Explanation
3. To begin with the practice of forgiveness, it is recommended to start with the enemies or people who have hurt us.	False	It is recommended to structure the practice of forgiveness in the following order: (1) forgive yourself, (2) ask others for forgiveness, (3) forgive others and give compassion to enemies, and (4) forgive loved ones who have harmed us. Therefore, it begins with being able to forgive yourself since if we are affectionate with ourselves, it is easier for us to be affectionate with other people and thus come to forgive them. Little by little we move toward forgiving others, at different levels (loved ones, enemies, and people who have hurt us).
4. Healthy reperception is one of the most effective therapeutic mechanisms for negative events.	True	It's true. The healthy reperception consists of not over-identifying with the negative aspects associated with the event but rather focusing on the positive aspects that this situation may have generated. These positive aspects are always of two types: (1) learning and resilience and (2) helping others.

14 Homework

Next, we are going to present you with a series of tasks. As you already know, carrying out the tasks that we propose in each module is a fundamental pillar of this program. Remember, the more you know and practice, the more you can benefit from the online intervention. Therefore, in addition to reading, listening, and reviewing all the information that is included in each module, we ask you to put the homework into practice. Think of a toolbox that you go to when you have a problem. We are giving you valuable tools. Now you have to learn how to use them. And don't forget: The more time you put into learning the material and doing the exercises, the more you'll benefit from it.

In this module we ask you to perform the following tasks:

- Read the content of this module carefully, and review all the material it includes.
- Do the Formal Practice 1 "Forgiving Yourself" at the least once *.
- Do the Formal Practice 2 "Asking Others For Forgiveness" at least once *.
- Do the Formal Practice 3 "Forgive Others and Give Compassion to Enemies" at least once*.
- Do the recapitulation practice (optional).
- Keep in mind the Informal Practice 1 of interdependence in your day-to-day life, and do it several times with objects and with yourself.
- Review and perform informal compassion practices in your daily life following the instructions in the Informal Practice 2.
- Use the Compassion Practice Journal to record your meditative practice on a daily basis.

- Keep practicing the Formal Practice "Compassionate Breathing" and "Compassionate Body Scan" at least once a week each.
- Review any previous module that you have questions about.
- Do any task/exercise/meditation that we have recommended and you have not done yet.

* *Note*: Depending on your situation, we recommend doing the formal practices of this module several times a week on alternate days.

Congratulations!! You have completed Module 6 "Understanding the Importance of Forgiveness."

In this module you have delved into the concept of forgiveness with the aim that you can be more compassionate toward yourself and toward others.

We encourage you to continue practicing everything you have seen in this module. Keep going; you're almost done with the intervention!

If you want, you can find the module summary in Annex 4.

You can also download the audio of the formal practices of this module.

Annexes of the Module 6

Annex 1. Formal Practice of Forgiving Yourself

Begin by adopting your usual meditation posture. Take some conscious breaths and feel your body as a whole. Breathe in and out, becoming aware of your bodily sensations. If at any time the practice seems too intense, you can return with full attention to the breath or the body.

Start by doing a general review of your life. Think of the times when you have caused harm to yourself or someone else, either consciously or unconsciously. These may be situations where you didn't treat yourself or others well. It could have been a time when you had too many demands on you and you were critical of yourself. Or perhaps not taking care of yourself enough. Or engaging in behaviors that weren't appropriate or consistent with your values and perhaps caused pain. Stay for a few seconds thinking of these moments.

Now, pick the one time when you did something that caused yourself harm (e.g., engaged in self-criticism or caused yourself pain), and reimagine the scenario. Don't choose the most intense event in your life but one that makes you feel a mild to moderate level of discomfort for you. It's ok if you don't remember every detail, but try to remember the event in a general way. When imagining this situation, place your palms facing up as a sign of acceptance, or perform the compassionate gesture that you feel most comfortable doing. While doing this, you can repeat the phrase: "For this time that I've caused harm to myself, consciously or unconsciously, I forgive myself." Repeat again: "For this time that I've done something that's caused harm to myself, consciously or unconsciously, I ask myself for forgiveness." Use the compassionate phrases that you would like while re-experiencing this situation.

Stay for a few moments feeling merged with this feeling of forgiveness, well-being, and affection that you feel for yourself.

Little by little turn your attention back to your breath and your body. Linger for a few moments, letting your attention rest on the natural flow of your breath, letting go of thoughts, emotions or images that appeared during the practice. When ready, you can return to your body, move your arms and legs, open your eyes, and end the practice.

Annex 2. Formal Practice "Asking Others for Forgiveness"

Adopt a comfortable meditation posture. Do a few conscious breaths and feel your body as a whole. If at some moments the practice seems too intense, focus on your breath or your body.

Start by doing a general review of your life. Think of the people whom you may have hurt, either consciously or unconsciously. You may be surprised by the number. The act of remembering them may cause you pain, but try to observe it without judging it and accept the experience as it is.

The feeling of guilt or discomfort may be intense. This may be because of the number of people who were hurt or because we have hurt those who are very dear to us. For some people, we may never be able to repair our actions. For example, the person might have passed away, or maybe you can't see them again for other reasons. In some cases, we may have done harm knowingly. This may be because we were also suffering and that pain led us to do things that caused harm. In other cases, we may have been trying to make the best of things, but it ended up doing harm. There can be many reasons.

Pick one person who you may have hurt. Spend a few seconds thinking about that person. Now ask for that person's forgiveness. You can use a phrase like: "I know I may have hurt you, consciously or unconsciously, and I ask for your forgiveness." If you have a mental image or memory of the person you've caused pain, you can imagine hugging them, if this feels comfortable to you, and saying, "I ask for your forgiveness." Take a minute and repeat the exercise with two or three people with whom you feel you've had the most conflict. If it feels comfortable to you, imagine hugging them, asking for forgiveness or telling them what you feel is appropriate. When you're finished, you can send them all your love saying things like, "I wish you well! I hope you can be happy! I wish you peace!"

If you start to feel uncomfortable or difficult emotions, turn your attention back to your breath and your body. When the emotion has subsided (which often happens when we focus on our body or breath), you can give yourself affection, because you are suffering in this moment. When you're ready, take some conscious breaths, feel your body in its entirety, and open your eyes, ending the practice.

Annex 3. Formal Practice of Forgiving Others and Giving Compassion to Enemies

Sit in your usual meditation posture. Take some conscious breaths and feel your body as a whole. If at some point the practice feels too intense, return to your breath or body.

Start by doing a general review of your life. Think of the main people who have caused you harm. Remember that thinking of this may cause you more pain, but try not to lose yourself in judging the situation, like thinking, "I didn't deserve it, why did they behave like this with me?", etc. Just try to feel whatever arises and accept it. Now select, two or three people who have hurt you in some way. Choose people who you feel capable of forgiving, without it being too overwhelming emotionally. Start with the first person you want to focus on.

Recall the situation: what happened, what did the other person do, what did you do, etc. Pay attention to the emotion that you feel when thinking of this situation, and try to name it. Think about how people, including the person who hurt you, are shaped by their history and their previous experiences. Your past and your history may also explain some of the ways you've hurt others as well. As humans, we're all pursuing the universal goal of being happy and free from suffering. Often, we can see how other people are trying to achieve happiness by taking certain actions, even if it harms us, or we don't understand it, and we don't like it. It's possible that the person who hurt you did it because they didn't have the resources, wisdom, or ability to act in a different way. Maybe they meant well, or maybe their own suffering blinded them to the hurt they were causing you. You may have done similar things at other times in the past.

Stay for a few moments, seeing if you can have a feeling of forgiveness toward this person. If you're not capable of forgiving this person, accept it, and mentally say the following phrase: "Maybe, in time I can forgive you, but now the pain is too great and I'm not capable of it." If, on the other hand, you are prepared to forgive without internal conflict, repeat to yourself: "Even though you have hurt me, consciously or unconsciously, I forgive you." Take a minute with this person. Only if it feels appropriate and you feel ready, you can imagine hugging them or showing them affection in a way that feels appropriate. You can also send well wishes to them using the following phrases: "I hope everything goes well for you! Hope you can be happy! May you achieve peace!"

Follow the same steps, with the second and third person that you have chosen. If you experience difficult or overwhelming feelings, redirect your attention to your breath, and let go of any sensations and thoughts. When the emotion has subsided (which often happens when focusing on your breath or body), give affection to yourself for suffering in this moment.

Finally, congratulate yourself with affection for having been able to carry out the practice, regardless of how far you've been able to go. When you're ready, take a few conscious breaths, feel your body in its entirety, and open your eyes ending the practice.

Annex 4. Summary of the Module

Objectives of the Module

- Deepen your understanding of what forgiveness is.
- Understand the concept of forgiveness and its phases.
- Learn how to structure the practice of forgiveness.
- Reflect on the importance and the usefulness of forgiveness to yourself and to others.
- Practice forgiveness toward yourself and toward others.
- Understand the things that can make it hard to forgive.
- Learn the main resources to help you forgive.
- Understand the suffering of others and give them affection, so you can start to do it in everyday life.

Module Contents

The Concept of Forgiveness

A common challenge that many individuals face with forgiveness is that many have been raised based on their family backgrounds or religions to view forgiveness as an "obligation." In this intervention, we view forgiveness as a choice rather than an obligation.

What Forgiveness Is Not

- Forgiveness does not imply that justice is not done.
- To forgive is not to deny the damage.
- Forgiving does not imply forgetting.
- Forgiving is not an immediate process but a progressive one.
- Forgiving is not an obligation, but it is always a voluntary process.
- Forgiveness does not imply reconciliation.

Forgiveness and Justice

Humans base interpersonal relationships on reciprocity. Generating harm to another person breaks reciprocity and usually requires some sort to repair.

The Usefulness of Forgiveness

Forgiveness is a very useful behavior both on a social level (improves relationships and cohesion) and on an individual level (reduces diseases development associated with chronic stress produced by sustained hatred).

Phases of Forgiveness

There are four phases in forgiveness to reach acceptance:

1. Recognition

2. Responsibility
3. Expression
4. Recreation

How to Structure the Practice of Forgiveness

We recommend structuring the practice of forgiveness in the following order:

- Forgive yourself
- Ask others for forgiveness.
- Forgive others and give compassion to enemies.
- Forgive loved ones who have harmed you.

Resources to Use to Generate Forgiveness

The most useful resources for developing forgiveness are:

- Recognizing the limited freedom in human behavior
- Dealing with perceived injustice
- Healthy reperception

Homework

Read carefully the content of this module, and check all the material it includes.

- Read the content of this module carefully, and review all the material it includes.
- Do the Formal Practice 1 "Forgiving Yourself" at the least once *.
- Do the Formal Practice 2 "Asking Others For Forgiveness" at least once *.
- Do the Formal Practice 3 "Forgive Others and Give Compassion to Enemies" at least once*.
- Do the recapitulation practice (optional).
- Keep in mind the Informal Practice 1 of interdependence in your day-to-day life, and do it several times with objects and with yourself.
- Review and perform informal compassion practices in your daily life following the instructions in the Informal Practice 2.
- Use the Compassion Practice Journal to record your meditative practice on a daily basis.
- Keep practicing the Formal Practice of "Compassionate Breathing" and "Compassionate Body Scan" at least once a week each.
- Review any previous module that you have questions about.
- Do any task/exercise/meditation that we have recommended and you have not done yet.

Chapter 9
Module 7: Consolidating the Practice of Compassion

Module Objectives

In this module, we want to help you achieve the following goals:

– Reflect on how you can have compassion for three different perspectives across your life history: your current self, your childhood self, and your parents.
– Identify and recognize the usefulness and importance of becoming your own attachment figure.
– Reflect and practice the emotional management of difficulties in relationships.
– Reflect and work on the concept of envy.
– Consolidate the practice of compassion and reflect on how to keep the practice throughout your life.
– Learn the importance of values and their relationship with compassion.

Go ahead with the module. Don't feel like you need to hurry through it. It's more important to try to understand all the concepts that are presented and practice the exercises.

Module Contents

1. Work in Three Perspectives
2. Usefulness of Being Our Own Attachment Figure
3. Formal Practice 1: Becoming Our Own Attachment Figure
4. Difficulties in Relationships
5. Formal Practice 2: Managing Emotions that Could Create Challenges in Relationships
6. Envy
7. Formal Practice 3: Work with the Feeling of Envy and Develop Joy for the Success of Others
8. Informal Practice 1: Changing Your Perspective

Supplementary Information The online version contains supplementary material available at https://doi.org/10.1007/978-3-031-38032-7_9.

J. García-Campayo et al., *The Attachment-Based Compassion Therapy*,
https://doi.org/10.1007/978-3-031-38032-7_9

9. How to Maintain the Practice of Compassion Throughout Your Life
10. Informal Practice 2: Our Values and Their Relation to Compassion
11. Exercise and Final Reflection: What Would Our Life be Like if We Started Over?
12. Self-Assessment Questions
13. Homework
14. Annexes of the Module

In this module, we describe how you can have compassion for three different perspectives across your life history: your current self, your childhood self, and your parents/caregivers. We will show you how you can become your own attachment figure. We also discuss how to deal with difficulties in relationships, and introduce the concept of envy. There are formal practices that go along with each of these components. Finally, we will go over how to maintain the practice of compassion throughout your life. Informal practices include changing your perspective as well as reflecting on your values and their relationship with compassion.

1 Work in Three Perspectives

The way you relate to yourself and to others does not just happen randomly or out of nowhere. It develops from our early experiences as children and the way we functioned as children, developed from our caregiver's own attachment pattern and way of relating to others.

As we try to understand our patterns of attachment, change our style of interpersonal relationships, or decrease our destructive self-critical voice, it is useful to work not only on our present functioning but understand our childhood experiences. In moments of high stress and discomfort, we may react in a similar way as we did when we were children. We might also be influenced by the attachment pattern that each of our caregivers had, which serves as the basis for developing our own (e.g., we might copy our parents' attachment style, or we may do the opposite of what our parents did). How we respond to ourselves when we feel bad is largely influenced by how our early caregivers responded to us when we felt bad (e.g., attachment pattern).

In compassion interventions, the main practices focus on three perspectives: (1) How we react when we feel bad now, (2) How we reacted when we felt bad as a child, and (3) How our parents reacted in general and to us specifically when things went wrong. We can then focus on having compassion for our current self (e.g., self-compassionate pause), our childhood self, and for our parents who were trying to parent us.

In general, many therapies or psychological interventions (psychoanalysis is the best example) reach the conclusion that our suffering (or important parts of our suffering) originates in childhood and the relationship we had with our parents. There are people who get stuck there: rejecting or blaming their parents, which is often not helpful.

When we approach things with compassion, we aren't looking for people to blame. Instead, we're trying to understand why we relate to others and ourselves in the way that we do and to unravel the puzzle from the present to the past. Therefore, one of the core practices in this intervention is to write a letter to your caregivers. This can be a way to prepare you for the possibility of reconciling with them; however, it's ok if you're not interested in or ready to reconcile with your parents.

In short, when you do compassion practices, it may be important to focus not only on the present moment but, from time to time, to return to uncomfortable childhood experiences and your relationship with your parents to help better understand your own emotions and relationship patterns.

2 Usefulness of Being Your Own Attachment Figure

One of the characteristics of the attachment figure is that it is a real or imaginary person who constitutes the highest expression of wisdom and compassion. They have a genuine desire for us to be happy and to not experience any suffering. We feel that we can tell them anything, no matter how negative, because they will understand it without judging us.

Rather than relying on another person to be our attachment figure, we can actually become our own attachment figure. Although we may not have all of the wisdom and compassion (because no one person does), we can still be the person who desires happiness for ourselves and treat ourselves with kindness without judgment.

For some of us, this practice of becoming our own attachment figure can lead to a greater ability to love and accept ourselves.

The adult that you are now, in spite of your limitations and defects, can be an excellent attachment figure who loves you, that is *always* with you, and in whom you can trust.

This is the main objective of the formal practice "become our own attachment figure" which we ask you to try in this module but only if you feel ready. If you cannot do it now, then it's ok to have your attachment figure remain another person or an idealized figure. You do not need to force this process. You can try it in the future or never do it. The important thing about the attachment figure is that it works for you and serves as a reference. It is not necessary for it to be you.

3 Formal Practice 1: Become Your Own Attachment Figure

Next, you will find the audio and the transcription of the Formal Practice "Become Your Own Attachment Figure" (Annex 1).

If you feel ready to become your own attachment figure, we encourage you to try it now (Supplementary Audio 9.1).

4 Difficulties in Relationships

Human beings are social by nature, but human relationships are not only a source of pleasure and satisfaction but also a source of conflict and suffering. In all species there are disputes between individuals of the same species, often over needs such as food or shelter, sex, hierarchy, or territory.

In humans, the motivations are basically the same, although the expression is more complex. But what sets us apart the most from other species is the duration of the conflict. In other animals, disputes are ritualized (they always occur in the same way), and, in general, they are not too emotionally damaging for the participants, since once the fight is over, the issue is forgotten. In humans, disputes in relationships are not ritualized, and emotions such as envy, hatred, or a desire for revenge can emerge that can last a lifetime and even several generations.

Psychological and Physical Impact of Relational Conflicts

Neff and Germer (2018) developed a guide based on the theory of compassion that we can use when working with the feelings and the difficulties we may experience in social relationships. Our feelings can be layered, like an onion, and it's important to recognize all the layers.

1. Interpersonal conflict: This happens when someone takes an action (e.g., does something that we didn't want them to do) or makes an omission (e.g., didn't do something that we wanted them to do). Two types of suffering occur in interpersonal relationships (Germer & Neff, 2019a; Yarnell & Neff, 2013):
   (a) Disconnection: Feeling separated, distanced or rejected by others.
   (b) Connection (or over-involvement): Feeling so close to others that we suffer from their suffering.
2. Unsatisfied needs: This action or omission of others in addressing our needs makes us aware that there is a psychological need that has not been satisfied. Some of these needs are recognition, affection, security, etc. In short, to feel loved.
3. Soft feelings: When a need is not satisfied for love or security, it is like a painful wound. This wound results in "soft" feelings or emotions that make us feel vulnerable and may open up the possibility of getting hurt by others. These might be feelings such as sadness, shame, fear, loneliness, hurt, or helplessness (Simón, 2015). When soft emotions are not responded to with validation and empathy for

the unmet need, it can make us feel like we need to protect ourselves from getting hurt again. This can happen consciously or unconsciously.

4. Hard feelings: Often when we feel the need to protect our soft feelings, we develop hard feelings as a layer of defense or protection. These might be feelings that are easier for us to connect with or show outwardly. For example, we may feel anger toward others, when behind the anger may be sadness, hurt, or shame (e.g., soft feeling).
5. Consequences: We may then (consciously or unconsciously) punish or act angrily toward the other person (e.g., criticizing, yelling) or toward ourselves (e.g., ruminating, self-criticizing). In reality, these types of responses usually make us feel empty rather than satisfied. These responses can also result in long-term consequences, such as problems in relationships, difficulty connecting with others, and negative physical impacts on our health. For example, chronic hatred produces deterioration of interpersonal relationships and physical consequences (neuroinflammation theory).

We summarize the guide in Annex 2.

We feel these emotions produced by relationship difficulties from the inside out (e.g., unsatisfied needs → soft feelings → hard feelings → consequences).

The best way to deal with these emotions is generally to work in the opposite direction – from the outside in (hard feelings → soft feelings → unsatisfied needs → compassion). Here are the steps you can take (Fig. 9.1):

1. *Become aware of the "hard" feelings*: Becoming aware means connecting with your direct experience (e.g., the way you feel it in the body). Do not evaluate or judge (e.g., do not get caught up in the hard feelings, like hatred, resentment, a desire for revenge, or guilt for harboring these feelings). Simply observe the feelings and your urges to act on these feelings, even see the usefulness of these feelings (e.g., it helps to defend yourself when attacked, even if in the moment it's not as useful).
2. *Look for the underlying "soft" feelings*: When you acknowledge the hard feelings, you can progressively connect with other softer feelings. This is part of recognizing all of the layers of emotions that we can feel.
3. *Understand the unresolved needs that have been activated*: Once you feel the soft emotions, you can identify which of your needs has been unmet or hurt in the interpersonal relationship (e.g., need for acceptance, need for security, need for respect). Like everyone else, you will have needs, of greater or lesser intensity, that need to be met periodically. It is necessary to be able to know where your interpersonal wounds are, to become aware when they cause you discomfort.

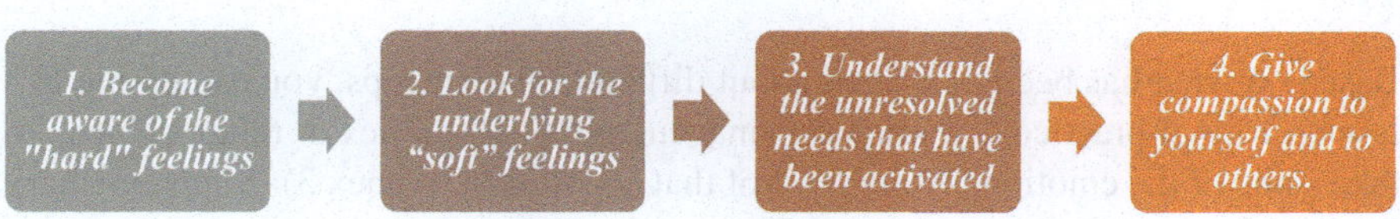

Fig. 9.1 Steps to deal with emotions produced by relationship difficulties

4. *Give compassion to yourself and to others*: What will heal that wound is the affection and compassion that you can give yourself. After you give yourself compassion, you can reflect on the characteristics of others, including those who have hurt you, and choose a new way of responding in your relationships.

You can make a choice to try to show compassion to a person who has hurt you as a way of handling the situation. However, you may not be ready to do this, and that's ok.

If you would like to try to show compassion to the person who has caused you harm, here are some strategies to connect with compassion for that person.

1. *Consider that people who hurt you are human and their actions are determined by their circumstances*: The person who hurt you wants to escape suffering and achieve happiness, just like you and any other human. Their actions are framed in this context. In addition, their actions are also determined by their circumstances (e.g., their history).
2. *Try not to use categories*: The categories of friend, enemy, and neutral person constantly change throughout our lives. In addition, they are subjective to each person. The person who hurt us has good friends and people who love him or her. If the person was "objectively" a bad person, everyone would hate him or her and, for most people, this doesn't happen.
3. *Recognize the usefulness of adversaries*: In Buddhist traditions it is said that adversaries help us achieve virtue and perfect patience. Therefore, we should value them because they draw our attention to our weaknesses and shortcomings (something that our friends don't usually do) and that can help us improve.
4. *Consider the importance of your own survival:* Hating someone for years has very negative effects:

   – On the psychosocial level: It can make you bitter, alter your interpersonal relationships, and prevent you from enjoying life and being happy.
   – On the physical level: It can facilitate the development of cardiovascular, psychiatric, endocrine, and oncological diseases by altering neuroinflammation factors.

Therefore, on a practical level, there is reason to stop hating those who hurt you for your own survival.

5 Formal Practice 2: Managing Emotions That Could Create Challenges in Relationships

Based on what has been described about difficult relationships, you can do the following formal practice "emotional management of difficulties in relationships" to take some of the emotional weight off of that experience (Annex 3) (Supplementary Audio 9.2).

6 Envy

Envy is an emotion of discontent and resentment that arises when another person is doing well, and you may even wish things would go badly for them. In principle, envy can appear in any relationship; it can take place not only toward people we do not like but also can appear when things are going well for friends and people we love. For example, this can happen when other people are doing well in a way that we want for ourselves (e.g., in a relationship, work, health, etc.) and we feel it is unfair that they have something we want/believe we deserve.

How can we not be happy that they are doing well?

There are usually two basic reasons for this:

- The first is a prejudice that considers that good things, the happiness that occurs in the world, constitute a limited good in terms of quantity. Therefore, if someone (even a friend) takes a certain amount of that happiness, it is less likely that we will receive it (e.g., there's a limited amount of happiness available; therefore a friend receiving happiness means less happiness for me). This magical thinking usually arises in the first years of life, in relation to our parents and siblings. Children have the idea that parental affection and attention is limited, and that they must be fought for against siblings. If parents listen to our siblings, it is likely that we feel less affection, and that is why we enter into competition. We can try to place ourselves in our first years of life and try to understand those feelings of childhood envy.
- A second reason, even more frequent, is the fallacy of justice: Many of us were taught to believe in a just world where if you put in the effort to do the right things, you'll be rewarded with happiness. As a result, we feel that it is unfair when happiness has come to another person when we feel like we've put in more effort and deserve it more. However, effort is not always guaranteed to result in happiness and we don't always get happiness as a reward for our effort.

There are *two lines of reasoning* that could *help manage envy* toward friends:

1. *Our happiness is unlimited and does not depend on other people or external objects*: Happiness is unlimited; therefore one person being happy doesn't make it less likely that I can be happy. This is like everyone being able to get an A in a class rather than only a certain number of A's available for the teacher to give.
2. *How does it benefit me that another person is unhappy?* Focusing on who is more deserving of happiness just leads to more suffering. Whether or not it is fair for another person to have happiness has no relationship to how deserving or likely I am to be happy. Feeling joy for another person, as well as ourselves, can increase our overall feeling of joy.

In the following information, we present the solution to envy: altruistic joy and empathic joy.

In the Buddhist tradition, there are four emotions considered extraordinarily positive: loving-kindness, compassion, equanimity, and altruistic joy or empathic joy. Over time, these emotions can often be achieved through the practice of meditation and compassion.

Empathic joy is a natural solution to envy. It involves rejoicing in the welfare of others, being happy when things go well for them, even if it's something we've been competing for as well, like a promotion at work, passing an exam, or dating someone we also like.

We can experience empathic joy for friends, but we can also feel it for people who are neutral to us and even people with whom we have conflict.

We can experience altruistic joy when we realize that happiness and well-being in the world is unlimited, that the "success" of others does not negatively affect us, but we can share in it because we are all interconnected. The happiness of others will positively affect to the entire universe, including us.

Like any state of mind, the emotion of altruistic joy is something we can learn to develop. It requires moving away from our usual egocentric and competitive thoughts and focusing on understanding the benefit that the joy of others produces throughout the universe.

7 Formal Practice 3: Work with the Feeling of Envy and Develop Joy for the Success of Others

Next you will find a practice to work with the feeling of envy and develop joy for the welfare of others (Annex 4).

We invite you to try it. If you're not ready, you can practice it at another time (Supplementary Audio 9.3).

8 Informal Practice 1: Changing Your Perspective

It's natural to think that, as humans, we are the center of the world. We might call this "personal importance." We often feel that the way people act toward us must be a reflection of how that person feels about us or is a reflection of who they are as a person. For example, when we get hurt, we may think the other person did it on purpose to bother or irritate us. However, people often do this as a way to avoid their own suffering and obtain their own happiness.

> When others insult us, lie, harm, ridicule, etc., we may think that they are purposefully trying to annoy or hurt us. However, people often do this for themselves, because they believe it will make them happier, and they don't know a better way to avoid their own suffering.

One informal practice that you can try if you feel hurt by another person is perspective-taking. If you think another person is targeting you because they want to hurt you, try taking a step back and consider alternative explanations. Do they treat others the same way? Is it possible they are acting that way because they don't know how to act otherwise or because they think these actions will reduce their own suffering? Asking yourself these questions can help you interpret others' behavior in a more objective way so that you can respond appropriately. This practice can also make other people's actions feel less personal to you and help alleviate your own suffering.

9 How to Maintain the Practice of Compassion Throughout Your Life

As we come to the end of this compassion intervention, we want to help you maintain the practice of compassion in your everyday life going forward. Here we present information on three topics related to maintaining the practice, including:

(a) Phases in your relationship with compassion
(b) Motivational foundations of compassion
(c) Values

(a) *Phases in your relationship with compassion*

Your relationship with compassion practices is similar to what develops with a partner:

There is usually (1) an initial infatuation phase, (2) a period in which the relationship stabilizes and the most emotional aspects disappear, and finally (3) it turns into either boredom or abandonment or becomes a stable, unquestionable part of your routine, and it's hard to go a single day without it.

Germer and Neff (2019b), in their training of trainers, describe practitioners' relationship with compassion as a three-phase process. As presented in the following Table 9.1:

(b) *The motivational foundations of compassion*

As for any change that we would want to make in our lifestyle or behavior, motivation is very important. The main motivational aspects that are related to the maintenance of compassion are (Fig. 9.2)*: insight, willingness, competence, immediate satisfaction, immediate reward, long-term benefit, and group practice.*

- *Insight*: The feeling that, with practice, you discover something new about yourself. It may be an insight about how you function in daily life or about how your childhood continues to impact you. Having that sense of self-knowledge and linking it to making changes in your life can be very satisfying.

Table 9.1 Three-phase process of practitioners' relationship with compassion

Phase	Description
Fascination and struggle	When we discover the technique as something wonderful, we are motivated to experience the fruit of our labor, so we try to practice exhaustively. It is like the initial phase of a romantic relationship
Disappointment	In a romantic relationship, one gradually discovers that the other person is not as perfect and they have their limitations and defects like any human being. Compassion, like any other practice, is doomed to disappoint. The reason is that most people use psychological techniques to manipulate the present experience and resist pain, which only produces more suffering. For example, if your partner has left you and you expect you won't feel pain and will heal immediately by giving yourself self-compassion, this is unrealistic. The problem is not the practice of compassion but the intention behind it. Disappointment is a natural and important phase of self-compassion training because it indicates that you are no longer trying to avoid pain but instead recognize it as an important part of the human experience. This is an intermediate phase
Acceptance	Acceptance is the last phase or stage (which is not always reached, as many drop out earlier). It is not about compulsively giving yourself compassion but about having self-compassion when it is needed and without the expectation that it will lessen the pain. As Germer says "we give ourselves compassion, so as not to suffer, but because we suffer" (e.g., we do it not to feel good, but because we feel bad)

- *Willingness*: Knowing that you've sought the intervention of compassion yourself instead of being made to do it by a professional, relatives, or friends. It is easier to sustain choices that are self-generated (voluntary).
- *Competence*: Feeling comfortable and competent in what you're doing (e.g., meditation). Doing the activity is not something artificial or foreign, and you feel you've developed and mastered the ability. In short, you can do it properly. Any activity where you feel a certain sense of mastery is more pleasant to do than those where you feel incompetent.
- *Immediate satisfaction*: The feeling of well-being produced by the practice of compassion in and of itself. In part (but not exclusively) it comes from a feeling of competence. When you experience satisfaction just by doing the practice, beyond the results obtained, you increase your intrinsic motivation to keep doing it.
- *Immediate reward*: When there is an immediate reward after doing something, it reinforces continuing to do that activity. If the practice of compassion gives you short-term relief, it will make it easier for you to continue practicing it.
- *Long-term benefit*: This type of incentive requires more maturity to recognize the benefit of doing something that can facilitate the change. Delaying immediate gratification (in the case of addiction) for long-term benefit is always tricky. In general, it's more motivating to think about the added beneficial effects (e.g., psychological well-being or quality of life, etc.) than the reduced negative effects (e.g., less anxiety and depression). Therefore, try to frame long-term benefits in a positive way (e.g., you're going to build something) rather than a negative way (e.g., get rid of something).

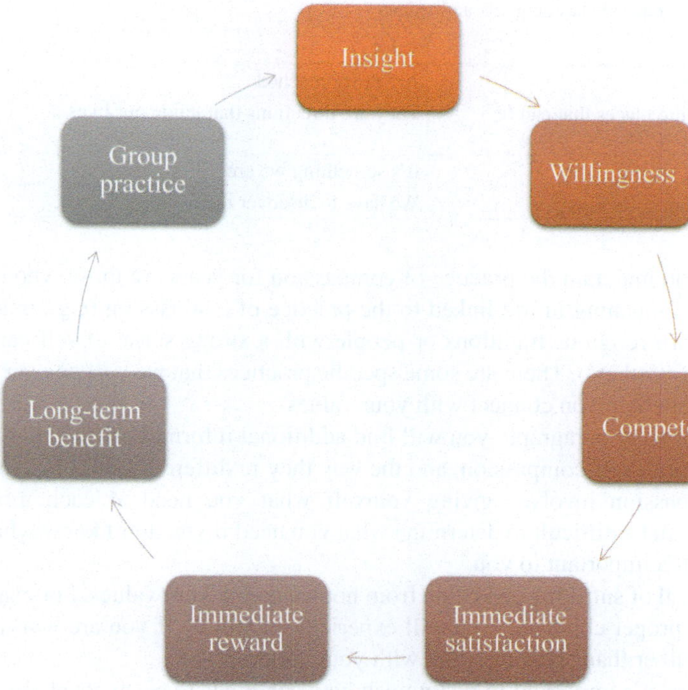

Fig. 9.2 The motivational foundations of compassion

- *Group practice*: This can be the biggest motivator of all. Having a group to practice with can help hold you accountable to keep up the practice, normalize your experiences, help you bond over shared experiences and training, make you feel part of a group, and make it easier to maintain the practice.

In short, changes in ourselves fluctuate over time, and we may not always experience steady progress. Each of these dimensions (e.g., insight, willingness, competence, etc.) can fluctuate independently. There are also other aspects that can negatively affect motivation, such as experiencing psychological illnesses (e.g., depression) or medical issues (e.g., chronic pain).

(c) *Values*

We're more likely to maintain an activity over time if it aligns with our values. Our values "are the principles that give our lives meaning and help us persevere through adversity" (Markway & Ampel, 2018, p. 28). Your values are how you want to say you lived your life (i.e., living your life by caring for people vs. living your life by trying to avoid pain).

It is important to review your values from time to time and think about the role that compassion might play in living out your values.

Table 9.2 Differences between goals and values

Goals	Values
Can be reached	Are never reached
They are specific places that can be reached	They are directions that guide our lives
It's something we do	It's something we are
We choose them consciously	We have to discover them

People who maintain the practice of compassion for years are those who have a clear sense of meaning in life linked to the practice of compassion (e.g., practitioners of Eastern religious traditions or people with a strong sense of self-care and compassion for others). There are some specific practices that we will go over in the next section, to help you connect with your values.

In the following paragraph, you will find additional information on values, their relationship with self-compassion, and the way they're different from objectives.

Self-compassion involves giving yourself what you need at each moment. However, it can be difficult to determine what you need if you don't know what you value or what's important to you.

A good deal of suffering can come from not following your values. For example, if you value proper childcare, you will experience suffering if you are working all of the time rather than spending time with your children.

In addition, it's important to distinguish between goals (e.g., to check on my ill father every day) and values (e.g., to be a caring daughter). Sometimes they get confused. The following Table 9.2 summarizes the differences.

10 Informal Practice 2: Our Values and Their Relation to Compassion

Here is a short and simple informal practice to help you explore your values:

> Close your eyes, feel your body and your breath, and imagine that you are at the end of your life. Ask yourself as you put your hand on your heart (or make some other self-compassionate gesture): What would give meaning to your life at that moment? Those are your values.

In Annex 5 you can find a template to perform the exercise including the instructions for the informal practice of values.

In addition, below, we provide you some guidelines that may be useful to you to reflect and get more out of this exercise of values, focusing on your values and their relationship with compassion. We encourage you to read it and apply them according to your case.

Are you removed from your values, from pursuing what would make you feel fulfilled in this moment? If you feel you are not acting consistently with your values, think about why this might be.

Think about if there are external causes (e.g., a difficult economic situation that makes it impossible for you) or internal causes (e.g., you are not motivated enough or you are afraid).

Try to reflect on whether with the practice of compassion you could gradually overcome these difficulties. If that's not possible, consider whether compassion might give you some relief from the pain of not being consistent with your values.

Think about whether your core value (e.g., helping people, being compassionate) can be expressed in the form of a vow or wish (e.g., I wish I could help people in this world). Once you identify this wish, you can recite it every day when you get up or go to bed. You can also try converting your wish into weekly committed actions (e.g., this week dedicate an hour to volunteering at a soup kitchen).

Another excellent way to practice your values is to make it part of your profession (e.g., finding opportunities to include compassion in the work you are doing) or as selfless help (e.g., in many volunteer organizations and disadvantaged environments there are ways to offer help).

Finally, another important aspect is to recognize that life is very long and that we all have periods of change. There will be times in your life when even well-rooted practices such as compassion will have less importance for you. Life is a long-distance race and all of us are going to have periodic potholes.

We encourage you to do this reflection from time to time, along with informal practice of values, to get the most out of this exercise. Don't forget to adapt it according to your case and situation.

11 Exercise and Final Reflection: What Would Our Life Be Like If We Started Over?

We end this compassion intervention with an exercise. Take your usual meditation posture, feel your breath and your body, and then think about what your life would be like if you could be born again with the experience you have now.

There are likely many situations that wouldn't change but others that would. Take a few seconds and reflect on the things that would change. Logically, you can't change your past life, but you can change the time that you have left.

You can think about your current life and how it differs from what your ideal life would be. You can always make changes in your day to day that guide you toward your values. What you have experienced with the practice of compassion can give you enough motivation to do so. Also, think about how the practice of compassion can connect you with your values, and vice versa.

Remember...

- In compassionate interventions, we're looking not for people to blame but for solutions. The goal is for you to understand why you relate to others and yourself in the way that you do and to unravel the puzzle from the present to the past, taking into account the three periods (present, past, and future).
- Becoming your own attachment figure can be beneficial if you can be the person who loves you, is always with you, and whom you can trust. This can lead to a greater ability to love and accept yourself. However, you don't need to force this process; it's ok to have your attachment figure remain another person or an idealized figure.
- Dealing with difficulties in relationships involves becoming aware of the "hard" feelings of hatred and resentment, looking for the "soft" feelings that underlie them, understanding the unresolved needs that have been activated, and giving compassion to yourself and others.
- There are two arguments that could help manage envy toward friends: (1) your happiness is unlimited and does not depend on other people or external objects and (2) how does it benefit you that another person is unhappy?
- The informal practice of changing your perspective can help reduce or alleviate your own suffering.
- Some aspects related to the maintenance of compassion practice throughout life are as follows: (1) phases in the relationship with compassion, (2) motivational foundations of compassion, and (3) values.

12 Self-Assessment Questions

You are doing very well! Now, let's review what you have learned in this module. For this, we will present you with a series of questions about the most important aspects. Don't worry if you don't know an answer; these questions are designed to help you.

Please answer the following questions:

	True	False
1. From the approach of compassion, it is only important to understand the causes and the people to blame for your suffering, that is why it is recommended to focus exclusively on the past.	T	F
2. Envy can appear mainly for two basic reasons: (a) the assumption that happiness is a limited good and (b) the fallacy of justice.	T	F
3. The relationship with compassion and its training is characterized by linear, constant progress.	T	F
4. Your values and the extent your actions are in line with your values are important for maintaining any activity.	T	F

Explanation of Self-Assessment Questions

Question	Correct answer	Explanation
1. From the approach of compassion, it is only important to understand the causes and the people to blame for your suffering; that is why it is recommended to focus exclusively on the past.	False	This is false. As you have seen throughout the module, compassion interventions do not seek people to blame but solutions. The goal is to understand why you function like this in the present, based on a review of past and present relationships but with a compassionate attitude of understanding that guides you to a future without resentment focused on improving your well-being. Therefore, it is recommended to work in all three periods (past, present, and future).
2. Envy can appear mainly for two basic reasons: (a) happiness is a limited good and (b) the fallacy of justice.	True	That's right! This is true. The first reason refers to the belief that happiness or good things constitute a limited good and the second is the fallacy of justice, or the feeling that we deserve happiness more than the other person.
3. The relationship with compassion and its training is characterized by linear, constant progress.	False	As in any learning process, learning compassion occurs in a spiral, so you will need to go through the same exercises several times to reach deeper and deeper levels of understanding. In addition, it is important that you remember the different stages of the relationship with compassion including: Fascination and struggle, disappointment, and acceptance.
4. Your values and the extent your actions are in line with your values are important for maintaining any activity.	True	This is true. For example, people who establish the practice of meditation for self- care and personal well-being (as a value or meaning of life) will be more likely to maintain the practice of compassion.

13 Homework

Next, we are going to present you with a series of tasks. As you already know, carrying out the tasks that we propose in each module is a fundamental pillar of this program. Remember, the more you know and practice, the more you can benefit from the online intervention. Therefore, in addition to reading, listening, and reviewing all the information that is included in each module, we ask you to put the homework into practice. Think of a toolbox that you go to when you have a problem. We are giving you valuable tools. Now you have to learn how to use them. And don't forget: The more time you put into learning the material and doing the exercises, the more you'll benefit from it.

In this module we ask you to perform the following tasks:

- Read the content of this module carefully, and review all the material it includes.
- Do Formal Practice 1 "Becoming Your Own Attachment Figure" at least once. *
- Do the Formal Practice 2 "Managing Emotions that Could Create Challenges in Relationships" at least once.*
- Do Formal Practice 3 "Working with Envy and Developing Joy for the Success of Others" at least once.*
- Keep in mind the Informal Practice 1 "Changing Your Perspective" in your day-to-day life.
- Do Informal Practice 2 "Values and their Relationship with Compassion."
- Reflect on how to maintain the practice of compassion throughout life.
- Use the Compassion Practice Journal to record your meditative practice.
- Keep practicing the different formal and informal meditations after the intervention is finished at least once a week each.
- Review any previous modules that you have questions about.
- Do any task/exercise/meditation that we have recommended that you have not done yet.

* *Note*: Depending on your situation, we recommend doing the formal practices of this module several times a week on alternate days.

Congratulations!! You have finished module 7 "Consolidating the Practice of Compassion."

In this module you have delved into the importance of being your own attachment figure, managing difficulties in relationships, the concept of envy, how to consolidate the practice of compassion, as well as the importance of changing your perspective.

We encourage you to continue practicing everything you have seen in this module. Congratulations, you've completed the intervention!

If you want, you can find the module summary in Annex 6.

You can also download the audio of the formal practices of this module.

Annexes of the Module 7

Annex 1. Formal Practice "Become Your Own Attachment Figure"

Adopt the meditation posture that you usually use. Take several deep breaths, with attention, and let go of previous emotions and thoughts. If you want, you can place yourself in the safe place that you've already developed in other practices. That place where you feel protected and safe and where nothing bad can happen to you.

You are going to start trying to develop yourself as your own attachment figure. For this, please follow the steps described.

Step 1. Developing yourself as an attachment figure

Bring to mind the image of yourself with the maximum expression of wisdom and compassion that you can imagine. Think about how you want to visualize yourself physically (it can be the age you want), how you are dressed, and what environment you are in (you can use the imagery that you feel is more related to wisdom). That attachment figure, which in this case is you, is related to great affection and compassion with yourself. Your image conveys security and commitment, the genuine desire that you are well, that you are happy, that you do not experience any suffering, and that you are always well. You also feel that you can tell this person or attachment figure anything, no matter how negative, because they will understand without judging you. Stay for a few seconds imagining these characteristics and thinking how this is the attachment figure that you yourself would embody.

Step 2. Using your attachment figure (yourself) in the present

Now think of some negative situation that you have had in recent months (6–12 months). Reconstruct the scene as clearly as possible, feel the emotion that arises and give it a name. In this moment of discomfort, imagine your attachment figure - which is yourself with maximum wisdom and compassion – approaching and comforting you in a loving way. Identify what the attachment figure would do to comfort you and to make you feel better. What advice would you give yourself, what positive aspects would you take from the situation, what would your attachment figure tell you about yourself, etc. Remember that this attachment figure loves you and understands you unconditionally, does not criticize you, and accepts you as you are. Stay here for a few seconds experiencing that comforting situation. Go to your breath; let go of any emotions that you were feeling.

Step 3. Using your attachment figure (yourself) in the past.

Lastly, think of some negative situation in childhood, when you were between ages 6 and 14. Reconstruct the scene as clearly as possible, feel the emotion that arises, and give it a name (sadness, anger, fear, shame, etc.).

Connect with that moment of discomfort and imagine that attachment figure (which is yourself with maximum wisdom and compassion) is approaching you, that helpless child who is upset, who is having a hard time, and hugs you, protects you, and gives you the affection you need. Feel protected and loved. Feel that discomfort is diminishing.

Stay here for a few seconds, feeling all the affection that you can give yourself in each situation, both in the past and in the present. Make the commitment to use it whenever possible, whenever you feel bad. Little by little, when you're ready, open your eyes and end the practice.

Annex 2. Summary of Psychological and Physical Impact of Relational Conflicts

1. Interpersonal conflict: This happens when someone takes an action (e.g., does something that we didn't want them to do) or makes an omission (e.g., didn't do something that we wanted them to do). Two types of suffering occur in interpersonal relationships:

   (a) Disconnection: Feeling separated, distanced or rejected by others.
   (b) Connection (or over-involvement): Feeling so close to others that we suffer from their suffering.

2. Unsatisfied needs: This action or omission of others makes us aware that there is a psychological need that has not been satisfied. Some of these needs are recognition, affection, security, etc. In short, to feel loved.
3. Soft feelings: When a need is not satisfied for love or security, it is like a painful wound. This wound results in "soft" feelings or emotions that make us feel vulnerable and may open up the possibility of getting hurt by others. These might be feelings such as sadness, shame, fear, loneliness, hurt, or helplessness (Simón, 2015). When soft emotions are not responded to with validation and empathy for the unmet need, it can make us feel like we need to protect ourselves from getting hurt again. This can happen consciously or unconsciously.
4. Hard feelings: Often when we feel the need to protect our soft feelings, we develop hard feelings as a layer of defense or protection. These might be feelings that are easier for us to connect with or show outwardly. For example, we may feel anger toward others, when behind the anger may be sadness, hurt, or shame (e.g., soft feeling).
5. Consequences: We may then (consciously or unconsciously) punish or act angrily toward the other person (e.g., criticizing, yelling) or toward ourselves (e.g., ruminating, self-criticizing). In reality, these types of responses usually make us feel empty rather than satisfied. These responses can also result in long-term consequences, such as problems in relationships, difficulty connecting with others, and negative physical impacts on our health. For example, chronic hatred

produces deterioration of interpersonal relationships and physical consequences (Neuroinflammation Theory).

Annex 3. Formal Practice of Emotional Management of Difficulties in Relationships

Adopt your usual meditation posture. Focus your attention on your body and take several conscious breaths.

Next, think of a person with whom you have a difficult relationship, toward whom you may have difficult feelings. Think of how you would summarize this person's relationship with you. Maybe the person started out as a friend, but as a result of doing something, he or she became an enemy, or someone you don't like. In either case, the person may have done or not done something that caused the relationship to rupture and may have produced difficult feelings. Focus on the most important actions or omissions until you are able to feel the emotions you have toward this person (e.g., hatred, anger).

Stay here for a few seconds in the difficult emotions you might feel toward this person. Pay attention to where you feel it in your body, while avoiding making judgments about the feelings that appear (e.g., feeling guilty for having hate, working out how to vent anger).

When you can observe the difficult emotions without judgment, try to connect with the feelings that are below it. It's usually feelings of sadness, abandonment, fear, etc. Often, they are so painful that, in order not to feel them, they turn into hatred or anger toward others, but if you can connect with that pain, you will understand your suffering and that of others. Stay for a few seconds experiencing "the heart of sadness."

Next, connect with your needs that have not been met: the need for recognition, for affection, and for security. If the relationship has affected you so much, it may be because those needs were not adequately met in your early years as a child. Try to connect with that time of childhood and with the wounds that you suffered then.

Once you have connected with that pain, give yourself affection. Adopting the compassionate gesture that you like, say the following phrases of compassion to yourself, adapting them to the situation: "I hope I can feel loved," "I hope I can feel safe," "I hope I can stop being afraid," or any other that you consider appropriate. Simultaneously, send yourself all of the affection that you can while you feel that wound is healing.

In the end, if you can, try to send affection to the person who has caused you harm, while using the phrases of compassion that you like: "I hope you can be happy" or similar phrases.

Reflect on this process of generating compassion toward those who have hurt you. If it feels too difficult to send affection to those who have hurt you, keep giving affection to yourself.

Little by little, when you're ready, open your eyes and end the practice.

Annex 4. Formal practice of Work with Feeling of Envy and Develop Joy for the Success of Others

To begin, assume your usual meditation posture. Take a few conscious breaths and feel the body as a whole.

Little by little, bring to your mind a situation in which you have felt envy of someone, and you wish they had more of what they had.

Think about the reason for that feeling: Is it a person you consider an enemy? Is it a relative or a friend for whom you felt envy? Is it someone who it seems everything always turns out well for? Reflect on the reasons why you've developed this feeling.

Perhaps you think that the happiness or good luck that other people have is unfair because you deserve it more than they do, or you might believe that happiness is a limited good and the more good things that happen to others, the less you'll receive yourself. There can be many reasons. Try to identify them.

Do feelings of envy benefit you or the world? Do you feel that the world is fair or unfair to you? Spend a few seconds answering those questions and analyzing the causes of your envy.

All of us feel envy sometimes, especially if we have an unmet need, and we see this need being met for other people. It's human to feel upset by this. See if you can give yourself compassion for feeling this difficult emotion of envy and for the unmet need.

Now consider the possibility of being happy when things go well for another person, because you know that this positive state of mind will improve their entire environment and many other people. See if you can wish the well-being of as many people as possible, because it will benefit the other people in this world and, by default, you as well.

Try to do this not only with your friends but also with strangers and even people with whom you have a difficult relationship.

As the Dalai Lama says, if you can rejoice in the well-being of others, you will always be joyful, because it is much more likely that something is going well for others (since there are 7 billion people) than for you (you're only an individual).

When you feel that you've connected, even partially, with altruistic or empathetic joy, redirect your attention to your body and your breath, and gradually open your eyes, ending the practice.

Annex 5. Informal Practice of Values

Instructions:

- Close your eyes, feel your body and your breath, and imagine that you are at the end of your life.

– Ask yourself as you put your hand on your heart (or make some other self-compassionate gesture):

What would give meaning to my life at this moment?

The answers to this question indicate your values.

You can write them down (this will help you remember them, and you can see if there are any changes when you repeat this practice in the future):

____

____

____

____

____

____

Annex 6. Summary of the Module

Module Objectives

– Reflect on how you can have compassion for three different perspectives across your life history: your current self, your childhood self, and your parents/caregivers.
– Identify and recognize the usefulness and importance of becoming in your own attachment figure.
– Reflect and practice the emotional management of
– difficulties in relationships.
– Reflect and work on the concept of envy.
– Consolidate the practice of compassion and reflect on
– how to keep the practice throughout your life.
– Learn the importance of values and their relationship with the compassion.

Module Contents

Work in Three Periods

The way you relate to yourself and to others develops from our early experiences as children. And the way we functioned as children developed from our caregiver's own attachment pattern and way of relating to others.

In compassion interventions the goal is not to blame others or feel guilty. Instead, we're trying to understand why we relate to others and ourselves in the way that we do and to unravel the puzzle from the present to the past, taking into account the three periods (present, past, and future).

Usefulness of Being Your Own Attachment Figure

The main goal of becoming your own attachment figure is that the adult you are now, despite your limitations, can be an excellent attachment figure who wants happiness for you, who is always with you, and whom you can trust. You do not need to force this process; the importance of the attachment figure is that it works for you and serves as a reference. It doesn't need to be you.

Difficulties in Relationships

Dealing with the emotions produced by difficulties in relationships involves a series of phases: (1) become aware of the "hard" feelings like hate, envy, resentment, guilt, and shame; (2) look for the underlying "soft" feelings like sadness, fear, loneliness, abandonment, disconnection, and loss; (3) understand the unresolved needs that have been activated; and (4) give compassion to yourself and to others.

Envy

Envy is a common hard emotion of discontent and resentment that arises when another person is doing well, and you may even wish things would go badly for them. It usually appears toward people we don't like, but we can also feel it toward friends and people we love.

There are two lines of reasoning that could help to manage envy toward friends:

1. Our happiness is unlimited and does not depend on other people or external objects.
2. How does it benefit me that another person is unhappy?

The antidote to envy is altruistic joy or empathic joy.

How to Maintain the Practice of Compassion Throughout Life

Some things that can help you maintain the practice of compassion throughout your life include: understanding the phases in your relationship with compassion, incorporating the motivational foundations of compassion, and getting in touch with your values.

Homework

- Read the content of this module carefully, and review all the material it includes.
- Do Formal Practice 1 "Becoming Our Own Attachment Figure" at least once. *
- Do the Formal Practice 2 "Managing Emotions that Could Create Challenges in Relationships" at least once.*
- Do Formal Practice 3 "Working with Envy and Developing Joy for the Success of Others" at least once.*
- Keep in mind the Informal Practice 1 of "Changing Your Perspective" in your day-to-day life.
- Do Informal Practice 2 "Values and their Relationship with Compassion."

- Reflect on how to maintain the practice of compassion throughout life.
- Use the Compassion Practice Journal to record your meditative practice.
- Keep practicing the different formal and informal meditations after the intervention is finished at least once a week each.
- Review any previous modules that you have questions about.
- Do any task/exercise/meditation that we have recommended that you have not done yet.

Depending on your situation, we recommend doing the formal practices of this module several times a week on alternate days.

ABCT Glossary

Compassion "A sensitivity to suffering in self and others with a commitment to try to alleviate and prevent it" Paul Gilbert (2015).

Self-Compassion "Being open to and moved by one's own suffering, experiencing feelings of caring and kindness toward oneself, taking an understanding, nonjudgmental attitude toward one's inadequacies and failures, and recognizing that one's own experience is part of the common human experience" Kristen Neff (2003a). Self-compassion *is not* pity or sorrow, forbearance or making excuses, weakness, or selfishness (or sin), and it does not decrease the motivation for change.

Compassion-Based Interventions Interventions that help people use compassion in everyday life. These interventions are usually structured and have manualized protocols that include theory, practice, and exercises to help people develop compassion (and self-compassion).

Attachment Theory When caregivers are consistently responsive and soothing, a child develops a view of themselves as valued and confident and worthy of having their needs met by others. When caregivers are inconsistently available and/or responsive or when they are punitive or abusive, a child develops a view of themselves as unworthy and/or incompetent, and not valued enough to have others meet their needs. Thus,

J. García-Campayo et al., *The Attachment-Based Compassion Therapy*,
https://doi.org/10.1007/978-3-031-38032-7

experiences with caregivers throughout childhood promote long-standing, sometimes rigid expectations about how one will be treated by significant others and how the person views themself (Bowlby, 1973).

Attachment The capacity for affection and trust that we feel toward ourselves and toward other people.

Attachment Patterns Develop based on early childhood experiences with caregivers.

Attachment Figure Someone who has all of the characteristics you consider essential to your security and wellbeing. This is someone who you see as stronger and wiser and whom you can turn to when you're not feeling safe or when you're suffering. When you're developing your attachment figure, several figures can coexist at first, but eventually you should develop one figure that combines all the useful characteristics. This figure can be totally invented or created from existing people.

Figure of Affection Something or someone that evokes a feeling of well-being, calm, and security and draws a genuine smile to your face. It should be alive at this moment and can be more than one person, animal, or thing.

Pain It is inevitable, and we experience it because it is inherent to human nature, so we must accept it (here accepting does not mean resignation, it means accepting its reality without rejecting it, which creates a space for more functional and adequate responses). It includes the painful physical and emotional aspects produced by aging, illness, and death – both for ourselves and our loved ones. We also refer to it as primary suffering.

Secondary suffering It is avoidable. We generate it by not accepting the reality of pain (or primary suffering). It's what we tell ourselves and how we react to pain (or primary suffering). An example of this suffering would be after the death of a loved one (which is obviously going to cause us significant pain) to think that no one will ever love us as much as this person, that our life without that person will no longer make sense, and that we will never be happy again.

Self-Pity	To feel sorry for yourself and assume that your pain is worse than everyone else's pain.
Destructive Criticism	Identifies a problem in a way that is global, unclear about what needs to change, judges the person, has a disrespectful tone, and focuses on the negative aspect only.
Constructive Criticism	Identifies a problem in a way that is concrete about what needs to change, doesn't judge, has a respectful and friendly tone, and also includes the things that are being done right.
Self-criticism	Self-criticism is when we evaluate our own behavior and attributes, which often involves judging ourselves for our own weaknesses, errors, and shortcomings. Although constructive self-criticism can have a positive effect in fostering personal growth, a tendency toward destructive self-criticism is thought by some to be a risk factor for depression (American Psychological Association - https://dictionary.apa.org/self-criticism).
Self-critical voice	When we criticize ourselves, speak in a very harsh tone or insult ourselves and, in extreme cases, blame ourselves.
Formal Practice	Involves selecting a specific predetermined place and time to practice/meditate (e.g., Tuesdays and Thursdays from 8:00p.m. to 8:30p.m.), using a specific practice or technique (e.g., compassionate breathing, compassionate body scan, etc.).
Informal Practice	Does not have a specific time but is carried out at any time of the day or in dead times (e.g., in line at the supermarket, in the bathroom, on the street, etc.), during day-to-day activities, but with a particular attitude of attention and kindness.
Mindfulness	the act of consciously focusing the mind on the present moment, being aware of any thoughts, emotions, or sensations that arise for you. Mindfulness is the opposite of automatic, habitual, or rote behavior and activity. When mindful, we are alert and awake, actively observing everything in our environment. Mindfulness doesn't mean rigidly clinging to the present moment, as if clinging hard enough would keep the present moment from chang-

ing. When mindful, we are open to the fluidity of each moment as it arises and falls away. Each moment is a new beginning, a new and unique moment in time. Mindfulness also doesn't mean rejecting, suppressing, blocking, or avoiding the present moment. Instead, when we're mindful, we enter into each moment (Marsha Linehan, 2014, DBT Skills Training Manual).

Meditation There are different definitions of meditation based on different traditions. In Zen, for example, one is often given the instruction "Watch your mind." In other traditions, one may be given words, texts, or objects to focus the mind on. This protocol will be referring to meditation as the secular formal practice of mindfulness, or practicing the skill of attending to, gazing, watching, or contemplating something while sitting or standing quietly for a period of time (Linehan, 2014).

Guilt An emotion that tells us that we have done something that goes against our moral code, such as the belief that we shouldn't hurt people. Ex. "I did something I shouldn't have done." "I shouldn't have done that bad thing."

Shame An emotion that lets us know that we are acting in ways or have characteristics that are inconsistent with the values and norms of our community. Shame is an emotion that serves to incentivize people to maintain the norms of the community. Ex. "I am something bad that I shouldn't be." "I am a bad person."

Hatred Extreme dislike of someone/something (Oxford Dictionary).

Gratitude Quality of being thankful, readiness to show appreciation for and to return kindness (Oxford Dictionary).

Empathy The ability to feel and understand the emotions of the other person.

Emotional Contagion when we experience the same emotions as another person, but in an involuntary way, and emotionally merge with that person.

Sympathy refers to the emotion you feel for another person, specifically the feeling of concern for the other person.

Altruism A helping behavior that benefits others, even though it could be harmful to oneself.

Altruistic Joy The realization that happiness and well-being in the world is unlimited, that the "success" of others does not negatively affect us, but we can share in it because we are all interconnected.

Empathic Joy Rejoicing in the welfare of others and being happy when things go well for them. We can experience empathic joy even if it's something we've been competing for as well, like a promotion at work, passing an exam, or dating someone we also like.

Soft Feelings Feelings such as sadness, shame, fear, loneliness, hurt, and helplessness that emerge when a need is not satisfied for love or security. These feelings often make us feel vulnerable and may open up the possibility of getting hurt by others. When these feelings are not responded to with validation and empathy for the unmet need, it can make us feel like we need to protect ourselves from getting hurt again. This can happen consciously or unconsciously.

Hard Feelings Feelings such as anger, hatred, or resentment that we develop as a layer of defense or protection when we feel the need to protect our soft feelings. These might be feelings that are easier for us to connect with or show outwardly. For example, we may feel anger toward others, when behind the anger may be sadness, hurt, or shame (e.g., soft feeling).

Self-esteem The appreciation or consideration of oneself and is based on self-evaluation, in the search for personal success, and continuous social comparisons to check that we are not "below" others in the qualities that we are measuring.

Loving-kindness A feeling of selfless love toward others (without attachment, without seeking personal gain) and reflects the desire that everyone be blissful and happy (Dalai Lama, 1997).

Forgiveness An individual, voluntary internal process of letting go of feelings and thoughts of resentment, bitterness, anger, and the need for vengeance and retribution toward someone who we believe has wronged us, including ourselves (https://positivepsychology.com/forgiveness-benefits/).

Envy An emotion of discontent and resentment that arises when another person is doing well, and you may even wish things would go badly for them. In principle, envy can appear in any relationship; it can take place not only toward people we do not like but also can appear when things are going well for friends and people we love.

Values Our values "are the principles that give our lives meaning and help us persevere through adversity" (Markway, & Ampel, 2018. p. 28). Your values are how you want to say you lived your life (i.e., living your life by caring for people vs. living your life by trying to avoid pain).

References

Allen, A. B., & Leary, M. R. (2010). Self-Compassion, stress, and coping. *Social and Personality Psychology Compass, 4*(2), 107–118. https://doi.org/10.1111/j.1751-9004.2009.00246.x

American Psychological Association. https://dictionary.apa.org/self-criticism

Austin, J., Drossaert, C. H. C., Schroevers, M. J., Sanderman, R., Kirby, J. N., & Bohlmeijer, E. T. (2021). Compassion-based interventions for people with long-term physical conditions: A mixed methods systematic review. *Psychology & Health, 36*(1), 16–42.

Bartholomew, K., & Horowitz, L. M. (1991). Attachment styles among young adults: A test of a four-category model. *Journal of Personality and Social Psychology, 61*(2), 226.

Berlin, L. J., Cassidy, J., & Appleyard, K. (2008). The influence of early attachments on other relationships. In J. Cassidy & P. R. Shaver (Eds.), *Handbook of attachment: Theory, research, and clinical applications* (pp. 333–347). Guilford Press.

Blackie, R. A., & Kocovski, N. L. (2018). Examining the relationships among self-compassion, social anxiety, and post-event processing. *Psychological Reports, 121*(4), 669–689.

Campos, D., Cebolla, A., Quero, S., Bretón-López, J., Botella, C., Soler, J., García-Campayo, J., Demarzo, M., & Baños, R. M. (2016). Meditation and happiness: Mindfulness and self-compassion may mediate the meditation–happiness relationship. *Personality and Individual Differences, 93*, 80–85.

Campos, D., Navarro-Gil, M., Herrera-Mercadal, P., Martínez-García, L., Cebolla, A., Borao, L., et al. (2020). Feasibility of the internet attachment–based compassion therapy in the general population: Protocol for an open-label uncontrolled pilot trial. *JMIR Research Protocols, 9*(8), e16717.

Castaneda, C. (2001). *Las enseñanzas de Don Juan: una forma yaqui de conocimiento* (Vol. 126). Fondo de cultura económica.

Castaneda, C. (2011). *El fuego interno*. Litoral, 251, 338–339.

Collado-Navarro, C., Navarro-Gil, M., Pérez-Aranda, A., López-del-Hoyo, Y., Garcia-Campayo, J., & Montero-Marin, J. (2021). Effectiveness of mindfulness-based stress reduction and attachment-based compassion therapy for the treatment of depressive, anxious, and adjustment disorders in mental health settings: A randomized controlled trial. *Depression and Anxiety, 38*(11), 1138–1151.

Cortés-García, L., Takkouche, B., Seoane, G., & Senra, C. (2019). Mediators linking insecure attachment to eating symptoms: A systematic review and meta-analysis. *PloS One, 14*(3), e0213099.

J. García-Campayo et al., *The Attachment-Based Compassion Therapy*, https://doi.org/10.1007/978-3-031-38032-7

D'Amico, F., Feliu-Soler, A., Montero-Marín, J., Peñarrubía-María, M. T., Navarro-Gil, M., Van Gordon, W., et al. (2020). Cost-utility of Attachment-Based compassion therapy (ABCT) for fibromyalgia compared to relaxation: A pilot randomized controlled trial. *Journal of Clinical Medicine, 9*(3), 726.

Dahl, C. J., Lutz, A., & Davidson, R. J. (2015). Reconstructing and deconstructing the self: Cognitive mechanisms in meditation practice. *Trends in Cognitive Sciences, 19*(9), 515–523. https://doi.org/10.1016/j.tics.2015.07.001

Dahm, K. A., Meyer, E. C., Neff, K. D., Kimbrel, N. A., Gulliver, S. B., & Morissette, S. B. (2015). Mindfulness, self-compassion, posttraumatic stress disorder symptoms, and functional disability in U.S. Iraq and Afghanistan War veterans. *Journal of Traumatic Stress, 28*(5), 460–464.

Dalai Lama. (1997). *The power of compassion: A Collection of lectures by his holiness the XIV Dalai Lama*. Thorsons.

Dalai Lama. (2001). *The Dalai Lama's book of love and compassion*. Thorsons.

DiBlasio, F. A. (1998). The use of decision-based forgiveness intervention within intergenerational family therapy. *Journal of Family Therapy, 20*(1), 77–94. https://doi.org/10.1111/1467-6427.00069

Fraley, R. C., Hudson, N. W., Heffernan, M. E., & Segal, N. (2015). Are adult attachment styles categorical or dimensional? A taxometric analysis of general and relationship-specific attachment orientations. *Journal of Personality and Social Psychology, 109*, 354–368.

García-Campayo, J. (2019). *La práctica de la compasión: amabilidad con los demás y con uno mismo*. ILUS Books Siglantana.

García-Campayo, J., & Demarzo, M. (2015). *Mindfulness y compasión. La nueva revolución*. Siglantana.

García-Campayo, J., Pereira, R. E., Melgares, M. L., & Moreno, S. P. (2004). Mobbing o maltrato psicológico en el trabajo. In *Actualizaciones año 2004* (pp. 153–168). Difusión Avances de Enfermería.

García-Campayo, J., Cebolla, A., & Demarzo, M. M. (2016a). *La ciencia de la compasión: más allá del mindfulness*. Alianza Editorial.

García-Campayo, J., Navarro-Gil, M., & Demarzo, M. (2016b). Attachment-based compassion therapy. *Mindfulness & Compassion, 1*(2), 68–74.

Germer, C., & Neff, K. D. (2019a). Mindful self-compassion (MSC). In I. Itvzan (Ed.), *The handbook of mindfulness-based programs: Every established intervention, from medicine to education* (pp. 357–367). Routledge.

Germer, C., & Neff, K. (2019b). *Teaching the mindful self-compassion program: A guide for professionals*. Guilford Publications.

Gilbert, P. (2009). The nature and basis for compassion focused therapy. *Hellenic Journal of Psychology, 6*(20), 273–291.

Gilbert, P. (2010). *The compassionate mind (Compassion focused therapy)*. Constable.

Gilbert, P. (2014). The origins and nature of compassion focused therapy. *British Journal of Clinical Psychology, 53*(1), 6–41.

Gilbert, P. (2015). The evolution and social dynamics of compassion. *Social and Personality Psychology Compass., 9*, 239–254.

Goetz, J. L., Keltner, D., & Simon-Thomas, E. (2010). Compassion: An evolutionary analysis and empirical review. *Psychological Bulletin, 136*(3), 351.

Gordon, K. C., Baucom, D. H., & Snyder, D. K. (2005). Treating couples recovering from infidelity: An integrative approach. *Journal of Clinical Psychology, 61*(11), 1393–1405.

Gu, J., Baer, R., Cavanagh, K., Kuyken, W., & Strauss, C. (2020). Development and psychometric properties of the Sussex-Oxford Compassion Scales (SOCS). *Assessment, 27*(1), 3–20.

Gumley, A. I., Taylor, H. E. F., Schwannauer, M., & MacBeth, A. (2014). A systematic review of attachment and psychosis: measurement, construct validity and outcomes. *Acta Psychiatrica Scandinavica, 129*(4), 257–274.

Hu, Y., Wang, Y., Sun, Y., Arteta-Garcia, J., & Purol, S. (2018). Diary study: The protective role of self-compassion on stress-related poor sleep quality. *Mindfulness, 9*(6), 1931–1940.

Inwood, E., & Ferrari, M. (2018). Mechanisms of change in the relationship between self-compassion, emotion regulation, and mental health: A systematic review. *Applied Psychology: Health and Well-Being, 10*(2), 215–235.

Jazaieri, H., Jinpa, G. T., McGonigal, K., Rosenberg, E. L., Finkelstein, J., Simon-Thomas, E., et al. (2013). Enhancing compassion: A randomized controlled trial of a compassion cultivation training program. *Journal of Happiness Studies, 14*, 1113–1126.

Kanov, J. M., Maitlis, S., Worline, M. C., Dutton, J. E., Frost, P., & Lilius, J. M. (2004). Compassion in organizational life. *American Behavior Scientist, 47*(6), 808–827.

Kirby, J. N., Tellegen, C. L., & Steindl, S. R. (2017). A meta-analysis of compassion-based interventions: Current state of knowledge and future directions. *Behavior Therapy, 48*(6), 778–792.

Krieger, T., Altenstein, D., Baettig, I., Doerig, N., & Holtforth, M. G. (2013). Self-compassion in depression: Associations with depressive symptoms, rumination, and avoidance in depressed outpatients. *Behavior Therapy, 44*(3), 501–513.

Krieger, T., Berger, T., & Holtforth, M. (2016). The relationship of self-compassion and depression: Cross-lagged panel analyses in depressed patients after outpatient therapy. *Journal of Affective Disorders, 202*, 39–45.

Lee, A., & Hankin, B. L. (2009). Insecure attachment, dysfunctional attitudes, and low self-esteem predicting prospective symptoms of depression and anxiety during adolescence. *Journal of Clinical Child & Adolescent Psychology, 38*(2), 219–231.

Linehan, M. (2014). *DBT skills training manual* (2nd ed.). The Guilford Press.

López, A., Sanderman, R., Ranchor, A. V., & Schroevers, M. J. (2018). Compassion for others and self-compassion: levels, correlates, and relationship with psychological well-being. *Mindfulness, 9*(1), 325–331.

Lopez-del-Hoyo, Y., Collado-Navarro, C., Perez-Aranda, A., Garcia-Campayo, J., Lopez-Montoyo, A., Feliu-Soler, A., et al. (2022). Assessing mindfulness and self-compassion facets as mediators of change in patients with depressive, anxious and adjustment disorders: Secondary data analysis of a randomized controlled trial. *Journal of Contextual Behavioral Science, 24*, 171–178.

Love, K. M., & Murdock, T. B. (2004). Attachment to parents and psychological well-being: An examination of young adult college students in intact families and stepfamilies. *Journal of Family Psychology, 18*(4), 600–608.

Luberto, C. M., Shinday, N., Song, R., Philpotts, L. L., Park, E. R., Fricchione, G. L., & Yeh, G. Y. (2018). A systematic review and meta-analysis of the effects of meditation on empathy, compassion, and prosocial behaviors. *Mindfulness, 9*(3), 708–724.

MacLean, P. D. (1990). *The Triune brain in evolution*. Springer.

Markway, B., & Ampel, C. (2018). *The self-confidence workbook* (p. 28). Althea Press.

Mikulincer, M., Shaver, P. R., & Pereg, D. (2003). Attachment theory and affect regulation: The dynamics, development, and cognitive consequences of attachment-related strategies. *Motivation and Emotion, 27*(2), 77–102.

Millard, L. A., Wan, M. W., Smith, D. M., & Wittkowski, A. (2023). The effectiveness of compassion focused therapy with clinical populations: A systematic review and meta-analysis. *Journal of Affective Disorders, 326*, 168–192.

Montero-Marín, J., Navarro-Gil, M., Puebla-Guedea, M., Luciano, J. V., Van Gordon, W., Shonin, E., & García-Campayo, J. (2018). Efficacy of "attachment-based compassion therapy" in the treatment of fibromyalgia: A randomized controlled trial. *Frontiers in Psychiatry, 8*, 307.

Montero-Marin, J., Andrés-Rodríguez, L., Tops, M., Luciano, J. V., Navarro-Gil, M., Feliu-Soler, A., et al. (2019). Effects of attachment-based compassion therapy (ABCT) on brain-derived neurotrophic factor and low-grade inflammation among fibromyalgia patients: A randomized controlled trial. *Scientific Reports, 9*(1), 1–14.

Moreira, H., Gouveia, M. J., Carona, C., Silva, N., & Canavarro, M. C. (2015). Maternal attachment and children's quality of life: The mediating role of self-compassion and parenting stress. *Journal of Child and Family Studies, 24*, 2332–2344.

Navarro-Gil, M., Lopez-del-Hoyo, Y., Modrego-Alarcón, M., Montero-Marin, J., Van Gordon, W., Shonin, E., & Garcia-Campayo, J. (2018). Effects of attachment-based compassion therapy (ABCT) on self-compassion and attachment style in healthy people. *Mindfulness, 11*(1), 51–62.
Neff, K. (2003a). Self-compassion: An alternative conceptualization of a healthyattitudetoward oneself. *Self and Identity, 2*, 85–101.
Neff, K. D. (2003b). The development and validation of a scale to measure self-compassion. *Self and Identity, 2*(3), 223–250.
Neff, K. D. (2011). Self-compassion, self-esteem, and well-being. *Social and Personality Psychology Compass, 5*(1), 1–12.
Neff, K. (2012). *Sé amable contigo mismo. El arte de la compasión hacia uno mismo*. Oniro.
Neff, K. (2015). https://greatergood.berkeley.edu/article/item/the_five_myths_of_self_compassion
Neff, K. https://self-compassion.org/why-we-need-to-have-compassion-for-our-inner-critic/
Neff, K., & Germer, C. (2018). *The mindful self-compassion workbook: A proven way to accept yourself, build inner strength, and thrive*. Guilford Publications.
Neff, K. D., & Seppälä, E. (2017). Compassion, well-being, and the hypo-egoic self. In K. W. Brown & M. R. Leary (Eds.), *The Oxford handbook of hypo-egoic phenomena* (pp. 189–203). Oxford University Press.
Pace, T. W. W., Negi, L. T., Adame, D. D., Cole, S. P., Sivilli, T. I., Brown, T. D., et al. (2009). Effect of compassion meditation on neuroendocrine, innate immune and behavioral responses to psychosocial stress. *Psychoneuroendocrinology, 34*(1), 87–98.
Pandey, R., Tiwari, G. K., Parihar, P., & Rai, P. K. (2021). Positive, not negative, self-compassion mediates the relationship between self-esteem and well-being. *Psychology and Psychotherapy: Theory, Research and Practice, 94*(1), 1–15.
Phillips, W. J., & Hine, D. W. (2021). Self-compassion, physical health, and health behaviour: A meta-analysis. *Health Psychology Review, 15*(1), 113–139.
Prior, V., & Glaser, D. (2006). *Understanding attachment and attachment disorders: Theory, evidence and practice*. Jessica Kingsley Publishers.
Raes, F., Pommier, E., Neff, K. D., & Van Gucht, D. (2011). Construction and factorial validation of a short form of the self-compassion scale. *Clinical Psychology & Psychotherapy, 18*(3), 250–255.
Rogers, C. (1995). *On becoming a person: A therapist's view of psychotherapy* (2nd ed.). HarperOne.
Santos, A., Crespo, I., Pérez-Aranda, A., Beltrán-Ruiz, M., Puebla-Guedea, M., & García-Campayo, J. (2022). Attachment-based compassion therapy for reducing anxiety and depression in fibromyalgia. *International Journal of Environmental Research and Public Health, 19*(13), 8152.
Simón, V. (2014). *Aprender a practicar mindfulness*. Sello Editorial.
Simón, V. (2015). *La compasión: el corazón del mindfulness*. Sello Editorial.
Steele, H., Steele, M., & Fonagy, P. (1996). Associations among attachment classifications of mothers, fathers, and their infants. *Child Development, 67*(2), 541–555.
Strauss, C., Lever Taylor, B., Gu, J., Kuyken, W., Baer, R., Jones, F., & Cavanagh, K. (2016). What is compassion and how can we measure it? A review of definitions and measures. *Clinical Psychology Review, 47*, 15–27.
Thomason, S., & Moghaddam, N. (2021). Compassion-focused therapies for self-esteem: A systematic review and meta-analysis. *Psychology and Psychotherapy, 94*(3), 737–759.
Tironi, M., Charpentier Mora, S., Cavanna, D., Borelli, J. L., & Bizzi, F. (2021). Physiological factors linking insecure attachment to psychopathology: A systematic review. *Brain Sciences, 11*(11), 1477.
Wakelin, K. E., Perman, G., & Simonds, L. M. (2022). Effectiveness of self-compassion-related interventions for reducing self-criticism: A systematic review and meta-analysis. *Clinical Psychology & Psychotherapy, 29*(1), 1–25.

Wei, M., Liao, K. Y. H., Ku, T. Y., & Shaffer, P. A. (2011). Attachment, self-compassion, empathy, and subjective well-being among college students and community adults. *Journal of Personality, 79*(1), 191–221.

Werner, K. H., Jazaieri, H., Goldin, P. R., Ziv, M., Heimberg, R. G., & Gross, J. J. (2012). Self-compassion and social anxiety disorder. *Anxiety, Stress, & Coping, 25*(5), 543–558.

Worthington, E. L., Jr. (2006). *Forgiveness and reconciliation: Theory and application*. Routledge.

Wu, Q., Chi, P., Zeng, X., et al. (2019). Roles of anger and rumination in the relationship between self-compassion and forgiveness. *Mindfulness, 10*, 272–278.

Yang, Y., Zhang, M., & Kou, Y. (2016). Self-compassion and life satisfaction: The mediating role of hope. *Personality and Individual Differences, 98*, 91–95.

Yarnell, L. M., & Neff, K. D. (2013). Self-compassion, interpersonal conflict resolutions, and well-being. *Self and Identity., 2*(2), 146–159.

Zessin, U., Dickhäuser, O., & Garbade, S. (2015). The relationship between self-compassion and well-being: A meta-analysis. *Applied Psychology: Health and Well-Being, 7*(3), 340–364. https://doi.org/10.1111/aphw.12051

Index

J. García-Campayo et al., *The Attachment-Based Compassion Therapy*,
https://doi.org/10.1007/978-3-031-38032-7

The manufacturer's authorised representative in the EU is Springer Nature Customer Service Centre GmbH, Europaplatz 3, 69115 Heidelberg, Germany. If you have any concerns regarding our products, please contact ProductSafety@springernature.com

Printed and bound by CPI Group (UK) Ltd, Croydon, CR0 4YY
30/09/2026
02225318-0002